Total Body
Shea Butter Recipes

Create Your Own Natural Sensuous Shea Butter Recipes
from The Top Of Your Head
To The Bottom Of Your Feet

G. CRUTCHER DUTCH

DEDICATION

This book is dedicated to the many
beautiful people who wish to maintain
their beauty with natural chemical-free
products.

CONTENTS

TOTAL BODY SHEA BUTTER RECIPES

REDISCOVER YOUR BEAUTY

Learn to make your own shea butter recipes. Not only will you be able to control what ingredients you do and do not want in your cosmetics, but you will also save tons of money creating your own natural chemical-free body butters. It's your body and these easy natural ingredient recipes will help you create your own body butters. Included are recipes to beautify you from the top of your head to the bottom of your feet.

Total Body Shea Body Butter Recipes
Introduction
Natural Skin Care Recipes
Benefits of Shea Butter
List of Natural Ingredients
Essential Oil Safety
Preservatives
Harmful Ingredients in Cosmetics
Recommended Suppliers
Recommended Utensils
Sanitizing Utensils Prior To Use
Have Healthy Beautiful Skin
Maintain Beautiful Healthy Skin,
What You Should Use on Your Skin:
Nice & Natural Hair
Prevent Damaged Hair
Fabulous Face
Mother Nature's Wonder Creams
Nature's Best Wrinkle Smoother
Eyes
Luscious Lips
Natural Makeup Remover
Natural Face Mask

Disclaimer

This information is not presented by a medical practitioner and is for educational and informational purposes only. The content is not intended to be a substitute for professional medical advice, diagnosis, or treatment. Always seek the advice of your physician or other qualified health provider with any questions you may have regarding a medical condition. Never disregard professional medical advice or delay in seeking it because of something you have read.

INTRODUCTION

If you think today's obsession with beauty is something new, think again! Ever since Eve took that first bite of the apple, humanity has been obsessed with beauty. Men AND women have been in touch with their bodies and beauty dating back as far as the ancient Egyptians.

Let's accept the fact: many of us are skin conscious. As much as possible, we want to have fresh, good looking skin. However, many of us fail to recognize that simple steps are the best ways to attain it. We tend to ignore what is right or wrong for our skin. We buy beauty products that tend to worsen whatever skin imperfections we already have. So, now is the time for change. We can do something ourselves to lessen most of those bothersome skin conditions we have.

This book will give you a look at natural chemical-free recipes, old and new, to help you meet the current view of our societal definition of beauty. You will be truly amazed and proud of yourself with the results from these age-reversing, simple beauty treatments.

In this book you will find general guidelines which are applicable for almost all shea butter recipes included in these pages. Making homemade shea butter creams or creating your own shea butter recipes is simple once you know how to add scents, how to melt shea butter, how to whip shea butter and how to store shea butter.

NATURAL SKIN CARE RECIPES

The skin is the largest organ of the body, it's also the first thing people see and one of the first things people base their impressions on. Why do you think celebrities shell out thousands of dollars to fix problem skin issues? Because their looks are their assets, celebrities will go to extreme lengths to get great looking, vibrant flawless skin.

I'm here to tell you today that you don't have to part with a fortune to get healthy, great looking skin. You can do it from the comfort and privacy of your own home and best of all, it's completely natural.

Healthy skin reflects our health both internally and externally. As we know the more natural a product, chances are the better it is for our bodies. The same is true for things we use topically. The less chemicals are used in our skin product choices the better it is for our health both internally and on our skin. Since our skin is porous, when we use things that are not natural, they seep into our systems causing toxicity and ultimately free radicals which cause cellular damage. There are many natural things we can use on our skin to help it stay in optimum condition.

BENEFITS OF SHEA BUTTER

Shea butter is one of nature's greatest beauty products.

Shea butter comes from oil extracted from the seeds of the Karite tree found in Africa. It is a luxurious, gentle, natural butter that stimulates the skin to make its own collagen. It offers some UV protection and makes a great moisturizer.

African Shea Butter contains a rich amount of unremovable fatty acid which renders it far superior to cocoa butter and other natural vegetable butters. This fatty acid is crucial to rejuvenating and moisturizing the skin. Shea butter provides all the essential vitamins needed to make skin look and feel smoother, softer and most importantly, healthier. Its therapeutic properties protect the skin from wind, cold, sun and it helps heal wounds faster. Shea butter stimulates cellular activity, fights the effects of aging and repairs tough, damaged skin.

The unique ingredients in shea butter also increase blood circulation to transport more nutrients to problem areas. This is extremely important if you have sun-damaged skin or your skin is showing signs of aging. It may also slow the rate of skin aging as it rejuvenates skin cells to soften wrinkles and fine lines and help skin retain elasticity.

Usage:
- Treatment of dry skin, eczema, and minor burns.
- Pain relief from swelling and arthritis.
- Improves muscle relaxation and stiffness.
- Great sunscreen due to its rich content of vitamins E & F. Vitamin F is especially important as its primary function is to repair and create tissue in the body.
- Treats dark spots, skin discolorations, stretch marks, wrinkles and

blemishes.
- Great when used for massages, diaper rash, and as a hair conditioner.
- Shea butter does not expire. Store in a cool place.

Many packaged beauty products that include it add poor quality shea butter and other unhealthy ingredients. You can save money and create a better product by making your own luxurious skin care products.

LIST OF NATURAL INGREDIENTS

Below is a description of the ingredients used in these recipes to ensure you that you are using the best natural ingredients.

24 Karat Gold Leaf
Pure gold leaf can promote skin metabolism, improves and beautifies the skin.

Almond Oil
Almond oil is derived from pure almond nuts. Almond oil restores and nurtures skin and is great for eczema and psoriasis. It's anti-inflammatory and keep the skin, hair and scalp soft and hydrated. Almond oil is especially helpful for people who have dry or sensitive skin. Almond oil is packed with vitamin E, which may help protect the skin from sun damage and premature aging.

Aloe Vera Gel (*Barbadensis*)
This natural gel comes from the juice inside the leaves of the aloe plant. Aloe vera gel possesses skin moisturizing properties and aids in maintaining soft, radiant skin. It is a powerful anti-aging agent and diminishes wrinkles, acne, pimples, age spots and blemishes and provides a flawless and youthful appearance to the skin.

Apricot Kernel Oil
Apricot kernel oil is obtained from the seeds of Apricots. Apricot kernel oil is great for use as a massage oil as it is very light and makes the skin soft.

Argan Oil (Argania spinosa L.)
Argan oil is a plant oil produced from the kernels of the argan tree which is widespread in Morocco. The vitamin A and vitamin E can help reduce fine wrinkles, it's a great skin toner, exfoliant for heels and elbows, and has been proven to reduce inflammation caused by acne. Argan oil helps prevent stretch marks, razor bumps for both men and women, is a great body moisturizer, helps promote hair

growth, and is a wonderful lip treatment that keep your lips soft, smooth and conditioned. It's also an ideal treatment for cuticles and nails, and dry, cracking skin on your feet.

Arrowroot Powder
Arrowroot powder is a white, flavorless powder comprised of starches extracted from various tropical tubers, such as the arrowroot plant and cassava. Arrowroot powder is used to absorb moisture. It doesn't have any antifungal properties, so it's used for moisture only. It is said to make hair softer, smoother, and less oily since it absorbs excess oil, it can absorb oil and dry out blemishes.

Avocado Oil
Avocado oil is derived from the pulp of the avocado fruit. Avocado oil not only treat sunburns, but also skin damage which includes dark spots created by the sun. Avocado oil can naturally encourage the rapid production of new skin cells. This helps to naturally resurface your skin's surface. Avocado oils do an amazing job of not only adding some much need plump to your skin, but it also traps moisture, which can help your skin repair from the inside out. Avocado oil will help to soften rough skin, while also leaving behind a trail of essential vitamins. This oil also works great as a natural hair detangler.

Baking Soda
In its natural form, baking soda is known as nahcolite, which is part of the natural mineral natron which contains large amounts of sodium bicarbonate. Baking soda can be used for minor injuries, including insect bites, bee stings, poison ivy, splinters, and sunburn. Baking soda can also be used as a natural deodorant, foot soak, detox bath, and exfoliator. Baking soda can help clear any clogging or excess oils that might lead to blackheads, dirt buildup, or even acne.

Beeswax (*Cera Alba*)
Beeswax comes from the honey comb of beehive frames. Beeswax is highly fragrant and completely natural and soothing to the skin. Beeswax effectively softens skin and creates a long lasting protective coating against the elements. Beeswax is anti-inflammatory, antibacterial, antiallergenic, and has germicidal antioxidant properties.

Bentonite Clay
Bentonite clay is clay formed from the ash of volcanoes. Bentonite clay is a natural ingredient that help balance sebum levels. This super-absorbent, clay has unparalleled oil-drawing capabilities that makes it excellent for oily complexions.

Benzoin Essential Oil
Benzoin essential oil is extracted from the resin of benzoin trees and is used as a tranquilizer as well as a relaxant to lessen tension and strain. In addition, use of this oil provides relief from tension, fretfulness, nervousness and trauma.

Bergamot (*Citrus aurantium*)
Bergamot essential oil is extracted from the rind of the citrus fruit. Bergamot oil aids in keeping the skin youthful, helps heal scars and other marks on the skin. It is also used to eliminate the unsightly effects of acne which can leave noticeable scars on the affected areas. Good for relieving stress and anxiety.

Calendula
Calendula is a genus of about 15–20 species of annual and perennial herbaceous plants in the daisy family Asteraceae that are often known as marigolds. The most impressive health benefits of calendula include its ability to speed healing, improve the appearance of the skin, lower inflammation, and it has great anti-inflammatory and vulnerary action, making it helpful with acne, ulcers, varicose veins, rashes, eczema and related conditions. It helps soothe sore, inflamed and itchy skin conditions and assists in soothing, and softening skin.

Castile
Castile soap is a vegetable oil-based soap traditionally made with olive oil. Castile soap may benefit individuals with sensitive skin and help improve skin conditions such as eczema and psoriasis.

Castor Oil
Castor oil is a vegetable oil derived from the seeds of the castor plant. it can help make dry, frizzy hair look smoother and shinier.

Cedarwood

Cedarwood essential oil is extracted through the process of steam distillation from wood pieces of the cedar wood tree. Surprisingly, cedarwood essential oil has anti-inflammatory, antispasmodic, antifungal, tonic, astringent, diuretic, sedative and insecticidal properties.

Chamomile Essential Oil

Chamomile oil is extracted from the flowers of the chamomile plant, which is a very popular flowering plant. Chamomile oil is known to diminish the scars, marks, and spots on the skin and on the face. Chamomile oil also helps protect wounds, cuts, and bruises from becoming infected.

Cinnamon Oil

Cinnamon is a spice obtained from the inner bark of several tree species from the genus Cinnamomum. Cinnamon extract can be used to slow the production of advanced glycation end products (AGEs), which cause wrinkles and amplify sun damage.

Citrus Essential

Citrus essential oil is a combination of orange, lemon, grapefruit, mandarin, bergamot, tangerine, clementine and vanilla.

Clary Sage Essential Oil

Clary sage essential oil is extracted by steam distillation from the buds and leaves of the clary sage plant whose scientific name is Salvia sclarea. One of the most well-known properties of clary sage oil is that it is an aphrodisiac, a substance or stimulus that has been said to boost libido and facilitate sexual desire. It tones the skin, muscles, and hair follicles, preventing hair loss and making you look and feel younger. Clary sage also functions as an antioxidant by tightening the skin that might be sagging. This oil has also been known to reduce skin inflammation and heal rashes. Furthermore, it balances and regulates the production of natural oils in the skin, reducing both oily and dry skin, making skin look young and beautiful.

Clove Essential Oil

Clove oil is extracted from the dried flower buds of clove (Eugenia caryophyllata). It has numerous medicinal properties and is used topically for pain relief. Clove oil uses are incredibly impressive, consisting of improving blood circulation and reducing inflammation to helping acne.

Cocoa Butter *(Theobroma Cacao)*

Cocoa butter is derived from the seed of the cocoa tree. This calming skin conditioner and skin protectant which melts at body temperature has a super-high mineral content. It is known medicinally to treat skin irritations. The moisturizing abilities of cocoa butter are frequently recommended for prevention of stretch marks in pregnant women, treatment of chapped or burned skin and lips, and as a daily moisturizer to prevent dry, itchy skin.

Cocoa Powder *(Theobroma cacao)*

Cocoa powder is fermented from the seeds of the cocao tree. It is a low-fat constituent of cocoa bean which is finely grounded. Cocoa powder's amazing benefits includes support for skin health.

Coconut Oil *(Cocos Nucifera)*

Coconut oil is an all-natural product made from the pulp of the coconut. It is excellent for moisturizing the skin. It's an anti-fungal anti-inflammatory natural moisturizer that is not oily and melts into your skin. Coconut oil is a natural sun protector which also softens skin and helps relieve dryness and flaking. In addition, it averts wrinkles, sagging skin, and age spots and promotes healthy looking hair.

Coffee Butter

Coffee butter is produced by hydrogenating the cold-pressed oil released by roasted coffee beans. Native women used it many years ago in their beauty regimen because of its antiseptic properties and healing benefits to the skin. Coffee butter is rich in antioxidants and great for battling cellulite, used in foot scrubs and foot cream.

Cornstarch

Corn starch or maize starch is the starch derived from the corn grain. Corn starch has been shown to possess anti-inflammatory benefits. It's soothing to itchy skin and calming to both rashes and burns.

Cypress Oil (*Cupressus sempervirens*)
Cypress oil is derived from the steam distillation of the branches of the tree. Cypress essential oil can help tighten up loose skin and muscles and prevents hair from falling out. Cypress oil has a spicy and masculine fragrance that can easily replace synthetic deodorants which boast a similar natural and distinct aroma. Cypress essential oil induces a calming, relaxing, and sedative effect on both the mind and body by relieving nervous stress and anxiety. It also stimulates a happy feeling in case of anger or sadness.

Distilled Water
Distilled water is water that has been boiled into steam and condensed back into liquid in a separate container. Thus, distilled water is one type of purified water.

Epsom Salt
Epsom salt, named for a bitter saline spring at Epsom in Surrey, England, is not actually salt but a naturally occurring pure mineral compound of magnesium and sulfate. Epsom salt has numerous health benefits as well as many beauty, household, and gardening-related uses. Epsom salt also known as magnesium is a naturally occurring mineral important for many systems in the body especially the muscles and nerves.

Eucalyptus Essential Oil
The leaves of selected Eucalyptus species are steam distilled to extract eucalyptus oil. This oil is antiseptic, insect repellent, and flavoring.

European Clay
European clay is a type of mineral clay with highly absorbent properties composed of a natural mineral silica. It's great for removing impurities, tightening the pores, toning the skin, exfoliating dead skin cells, reducing inflammation in acne and clearing skin problems such as blemishes, and black and white heads.

Evening Primrose Oil (*Oenothera biennis*)
Evening primrose oil is the oil derived from the seeds of the evening primrose plant. This oil is essential to keeping skin healthy and works well on dry and mature skin.

Extra Virgin Olive Oil (*Olea Europaea*)
Olive oil is a liquid fat produced by pressing whole olives from the olive tree crop of the Mediterranean Basin. Extra virgin olive oil, all by itself, is the best-known beauty secrets of ancient Greece. EVOO is a natural, hypoallergenic skin moisturizer that provide strong antioxidants like vitamins A and E that help repair and renew skin that has been damaged by modern-day environmental hazards. great for both your skin and hair.

Fir Essential Oil (*Abies balsamea*)
Fir Essential Oil is steam distilled from the needles of the Silver Fir, a tall, majestic evergreen that is indigenous to Europe. Fir needle essential oil can reduce pain, prevent infections, improve respiratory function, increase the metabolism, detoxify the body, and reduce body odor.

Fractionated Coconut Oil
Fractionated coconut oil also called "liquid coconut oil" is a form of coconut oil that has had the long-chain fatty acids removed via hydrolysis and steam distillation.

Frankincense Essential Oil (*Boswellia sacra*)
Frankincense oil is extracted from the gum or resin of frankincense or olibanum trees. Frankincense essential oil is used to relieve blemishes, dry and mature skin, scars, wounds, and wrinkles. It has been used medicinally for rheumatism, and skin diseases.

Geranium Essential Oil (*Pelargonium odorantissimum*)
Geranium essential oil is extracted through steam distillation of stems and leaves of the geranium plant. Geranium oil helps almost any skin type or skin condition. Its stimulating action promotes the regeneration of skin cells and speeds the healing of acne and blemishes. It also soothes dry, sensitive skin. Geranium oil imparts a healthy glow to the complexion, making the skin appear radiant and more youthful. It improves the appearance of broken capillaries and varicose veins. GEO also helps control excessive oiliness of the skin.

Geranium Rose
Geranium Rose oil is extracted from the leaves and stem of the rose geranium plant. Rose geranium tightens facial skin and slows down

the effects of aging, may help with any muscle cramps, aches and/or pains, has potent antibacterial and anti-fungal abilities. Geranium rose aids in eliminating bodily odors and can be used as a natural deodorant. Geranium oil can help in the treatment of acne, dermatitis and skin diseases, also inhibits the inflammatory responses of the joints. Geranium oil is commonly used as a natural bug repellant.

Ginger Essential Oil

Ginger essential oil is taken from the underground stem of the ginger plant. Ginger essential oil is an essential oil that works as an antiseptic, laxative, tonic and stimulant and anti-inflammatory agent. Ginger essential oil, is stimulating and therefore, relieves depression, mental stress, exhaustion, dizziness, restlessness, and anxiety.

Grapefruit Essential Oil

Grapefruit oil (Citrus paradisi) is extracted from the peel of the grapefruit. Grapefruit essential oil is known for its stimulant, tonic, lymphatic, disinfectant, diuretic, astringent, antiseptic, and antidepressant properties. Grapefruit oil's antibacterial properties may also have a positive effect on the skin, which could help fight bacteria that cause acne. Grapefruit oil could also benefit skin by reducing cellulite; healing wounds, bites, and cuts. The addition of grapefruit oil to conditioner or shampoo can help decrease grease and sweat and help the shine and volume of hair.

Grapefruit Seed Extract

Grapefruit seed extract, also known as citrus seed extract, is a liquid extract derived from the seeds, pulp, and white membranes of grapefruit. Self-made natural GSE processed in the laboratory without synthetic agents is prepared by grinding the grapefruit seed and juiceless pulp, then mixing with glycerin. Grapefruit seed extract encourages wounds to heal, excellent remedy for toenail fungus, and an effective natural preservative for cosmetics. GSE helps alkalize the body, useful for pets and can be used to discourage fleas and skin conditions.

Grapeseed Oil (*Vitis vinifera*)

Grapeseed oil is pressed from the seeds of grapes. Grapeseed oil contains antioxidants and anti-inflammatory properties, both of which are great for treating acne. The oil also contains linoleic acid, which is great for promoting skin health. It helps tighten skin and close the pores. In addition to these, it is a good remedy for reducing dark patches around the eyes and for skin rejuvenation (antiaging properties).

Ground Cinnamon
Cinnamon is a spice obtained from the inner bark of several tree species from the genus Cinnamomum. Cinnamon is used mainly as an aromatic condiment and flavoring additive.

Ground Nutmeg
Nutmeg is the seed or ground spice of several species of the genus Myristica.

Honey
Honey is a sweet, viscous food substance produced by bees and some related insects. Honey is all natural, with a host of health benefits and can truly be called a miracle food. Honey's super health powers are due to the multitude of nutrients it contains – carbohydrates, minerals, vitamins and amino acids. In addition, honey is antibacterial, anti-inflammatory and contains no fat. The natural antibacterial properties in honey has been used for centuries as a beauty aid and to smooth and soften skin, reducing the signs of aging. The natural antioxidants in honey make it a great anti-aging aid, while the antibacterial properties help to cleanse the pores. This helps to reduce acne and spots. In addition, honey naturally moisturizes the skin, giving it a youthful glow.

Hyssop Oil
Hyssop essential oil is extracted from the hyssop herb also known by its botanical name – Hyssopus officinalis. Hyssop essential oil's benefits and uses include feelings of alertness along with a reduction in fatigue and anxiety. Among its many therapeutic properties, hyssop essential oil can boast antiseptic, antiviral, antispasmodic, digestive, decongestant, anti-inflammatory, and pain-relieving actions. It can help relieve anxiety and ease the troubled mind.

Jasmine Essential Oil
Jasmine is a genus of shrubs and vines in the olive family. Jasmine

essential oil's benefits and uses include a floral fragrance that soothes, relaxes, and uplifts. It is beneficial for the skin due to its balancing nature. Jasmine oil can be used to reduce anxiety, stress, depression, and menstrual issues. It is also known to reduce skin issues such as wrinkles, eczema, and greasy skin. It can treat dry skin and improve elasticity in stressed skin.

Jojoba Oil (*Simmondsia Chinensis*)

Jojoba oil is a very popular liquid wax extracted from an American straw that grows wild. It is so close to our own skin that it's a wonder conditioner for skin. Keeps out drying agents on the skin and it is rich in vitamins A and E.

Kaolin Clay

Kaolin clay is a natural clay found in different parts of the world, and naturally produced by chemical reaction of aluminum silicate minerals in rock and soil. A Kaolin clay mask will thwart dirt and dead cells by exfoliating, and as a detoxifying agent. It will leave your skin moist and well hydrated, can sometimes be used for skin whitening. Kaolin clay mask cleanses dead cells and strips excess oil from the skin. Kaolin clay is anti-inflammatory and reduces acne inflammation, resulting in smooth and nourished skin. Kaolin clay help to remove dead cells and stimulate cell regeneration.

Kokum Butter

Kokum is mostly grown in the western ghat region of India which is known as the Konkan Region. The butter is extracted from the fruit kernels and is rich in antioxidants, vitamin E, and citric acid and is used extensively in dry skin therapies. Kokum butter is known for its antibacterial, anti-inflammatory and antioxidant properties. Can be used as a hair conditioner to make your hair soft and more manageable. Helps regenerate skin cells and is used to treat acne, dry hair, split ends and dandruff.

Lavender Oil (*Lavendula Spp.*)

Lavender oil is an essential oil obtained by distillation from the flower spikes of certain species of lavender. It is a mild oil with an easy, floral herbal scent known for its calming, relaxing and soothing effects. It can remove stretch marks and has anti-inflammatory, antibacterial, and bactericidal properties. It balances oil production, helps heal blemishes and stimulates circulation to the skin. Lavender oil reduces the inflammation of acne and soothes the pain of sunburn. It regulates the oil secretions of the scalp and helps repair damaged or over processed hair. Lavender oil soothes the inflammation of skin disorders, including psoriasis, eczema and other types of dermatitis. It cools burns.

Lemon Essential Oil (*Citrus limon*)
Lemon oil is made by cold-pressing the peels of lemons. The health benefits of lemon oil can be attributed to its stimulating, calming, anti-infection, astringent, detoxifying, antiseptic, disinfectant, sleep inducing, and antifungal properties. It could treat stress disorders, fever, infections, asthma, overweight, insomnia, skin disorders, hair disorders, stomach problems and tiredness. Lemon oil balances overactive sebaceous glands that lead to oily or blemished skin, helps clear acne and controls oily hair and dandruff. It revitalizes sluggish or mature skin and helps reduce cellulite by improving circulation and encouraging the elimination of wastes. Lemon essential oil encourages exfoliation of dead skin, enlivens the complexion and can strengthen brittle nails.

Lemon Eucalyptus Oil (*Eucalyptus citriodora*)
Also referred to as lemon-scented eucalyptus. The oil possesses numerous medicinal qualities and is often found in many products but is most commonly used as an effective insect repellent. And it can also eliminate fungus.

Lemongrass Essential Oil (*Cymbopogon flexuosus*)
Lemongrass essential oil is created by steam distilling the leaves/blades from this grass. It stimulates hair treatment, serves as a good room deodorizer and is also an insect deterrent. Lemon essential oil helps relieve pain in muscles, joints, toothache and headache, etc. It also helps cure body pain resulting from sudden exercises, sports etc. It is <u>not</u> recommended for use during pregnancy.

Lime Oil
Lime essential oil is produced by steam distillation from the peel of the fruit from one of two lime trees known scientifically as Citrus aurantifolia. The health benefits of lime essential oil include

antiseptic, antibacterial, antiviral and astringent activities among others. Lime oil also contains astringent and antioxidant properties that will help rejuvenate the skin. Lime oil can help alleviate feelings of stress and anxiety. Lime oil can provide excellent pain relief, relieve muscular aches and can help treat scalp issues like dandruff.

Macadamia Oil

Macadamia oil is a genus of a species of trees indigenous to Australia and constituting part of the plant family Proteaceae. Macadamia nut oil has several advantages for the hair and body. It takes on characteristics of oils like coconut, olive, and jojoba, making it one of the most versatile oils in your cabinet. It's health benefits for the heart, and the rest of the body is substantial. It's full of antioxidants, fatty acids, vitamins, and minerals. Macadamia nut oil contains a unique anti-aging ingredient, palmitic acid, which promotes the production of sebum.

Magnesium Topical Spray

Magnesium topical spray contains a 100% natural solution of magnesium chloride. It is extremely pure, mined deep under the earth's surface from the pristine Zechstein seabed in the Netherlands. It can be used daily, is non-greasy and has no odor.

Mango Butter

Mango butter comes from kernels of the mango tree. This butter provides protection against the sun, prevents skin drying, anti-aging and great to fight wrinkles, reduces degeneration of skin cells, and restores elasticity to skin.

Marjoram Oil

Marjoram essential oil is extracted by steam distillation of both fresh and dried leaves of the marjoram plant, which has the scientific name Origanum majorana. Marjoram essential oil is used in aromatherapy to provide a natural remedy for acne, eczema, and maintain skin texture when mixed with creams. It is used to massage the muscles, calm the nerves and to relieve stress.

Menthol Crystals

Menthol crystals is 100% Organic, All-Natural Menthol Crystals made from Peppermint Oil. Menthol has a refreshing and cooling effect on skin and is added to products because of its characteristic aroma, flavor, and numbing effects. It has the anti-fungal, antibacterial and pain management actions of Menthol.

Neroli Essential Oil

Neroli is extracted by steam distillation from a citrus fruit. The health benefits of neroli essential oil can be attributed to its properties as an antidepressant, aphrodisiac, antiseptic, bactericidal, disinfectant, antispasmodic, deodorant, digestive, emollient, sedative, and tonic substance.

Orange Essential Oil (*Citrus sinensis*)

Orange essential oil is obtained from the peels of oranges by cold compression. Orange oil restores balance to dry or oily skin. It maintains healthy, youthful skin by promoting the production of collagen. It reduces puffiness and discourages dry or wrinkled skin. Orange oil stimulates circulation to the skin surface and softens rough skin. It also clears blemishes and improves acne prone skin, helps reduce tissue swelling and fluid retention. It improves cellulite, which is sometimes called-orange peel skin.

Palm Oil

Palm oil is an edible vegetable oil derived from the reddish pulp of the fruit of the oil palms, primarily the African oil palm Elaeis guineensis.

Patchouli Essential Oil

Patchouli oil is basically an essential oil which is extracted from the leaves of the patchouli plant. It is an herb which belongs to the mint family. Patchouli is known to relieve depression, and soothes inflammation.

Peach Essential Oil

Peach essential oil is created from the kernel of their peach and used for its rejuvenating qualities and healing properties. It has high amounts of antioxidants that have significant anti-inflammatory effects on the body. Peach oil is an excellent skin moisturizer that penetrates quickly into the skin cells, thanks to its molecular structure. This essential oil is helpful in restoring nails that have been damaged by artificial nail treatments and it is used to soothe inflamed skin. It is rich in Vitamin C which helps your skin defend itself against inflammation.

Peppermint Oil (*Mentha Piperita*)

Peppermint essential oil is steam distilled from the fragrant herb; it is primarily composed of the chemical components menthol and menthone. Peppermint oil is used for acne, dermatitis, and as flavoring and fragrance in cosmetics. Peppermint oil fights bacterial infection and reduces the oiliness present with acne and blemishes. It stimulates circulation and helps enliven dull, dry skin. Peppermint oil leaves skin feeling soft and silky. It also regulates and normalizes oily skin and hair. It minimizes the redness of broken capillaries and varicose veins.

Pistachio Butter

Made by taking pure pistachio oil and mixing with other oils. Great butter for the skin, penetrates easily, does not clog pores or cause any irritation to skin. Exotic.

Rose Clay

Often referred to as pink clay, is a gentle, natural clay that contains kaolinite. Rose clay is fabulous for most skin types; including sensitive skin. Rose clay provides gentle exfoliation, helps to draw toxins from the skin, helps to increase circulation, reduces skin irritation, and helps to reduce inflammation.

Rose Essential Oil (*Rosa damascene*)

Rose oil is the essential oil extracted from the petals of various types of rose. Rose Essential Oil is used to relieve broken capillaries, conjunctivitis, dry skin, eczema, mature and sensitive complexions and wrinkles. It is suitable for all skin types, but it is especially valuable for dry, sensitive or aging skin. It helps restore the moisture balance and soothes wrinkles.

Rosehip Seed Oil

Rosehip seed oil is a pressed seed oil, extracted from the seeds of the wild rose bush in the Southern Andes. Rosehip oil can work as a great natural alternative for moisturizing. Rosehip oil is packed with beauty essentials like anti-inflammatory fatty acids and vitamins A and C. These ingredients allow rosehip oil to treat signs of aging and pigmentation, hydrate skin and repair damaged skin. The fatty acids and vitamins A and C make this oil a potential solution for fading any facial scars or unsightly marks.

Rosemary Oil (*Rosmarinus officinalis*)
Rosemary is an herb. The oil is extracted from the leaf and used to make medicine. Rosemary oil can encourage hair growth, increase mental activity, relieve respiratory problems and reduce pain. Its anti-inflammatory ability has been known to relieve pain in headaches, muscle pain, rheumatism, and arthritis. Rosemary oil stimulates cell renewal. It improves dry or mature skin, eases lines and wrinkles, and heals burns and wounds. It can also clear acne, blemishes, or dull, dry skin. Rosemary oil nourishes the scalp and keeps hair looking healthy and shiny. It normalizes excessive oil secretions and improves most scalp problems, particularly dandruff and seborrhea. Rosemary is also helpful in treating cellulite.

Sage Oil
Sage oil is made by steam distillation of Salvia officinalis partially dried leaves. The health benefits of sage essential oil can be attributed to its properties as an antifungal, antimicrobial, antioxidant, antiseptic, anti-inflammatory, antispasmodic, antibacterial, disinfectant, expectorant, laxative, and a stimulating substance.

Sandalwood Essential Oil
Sandalwood is a class of woods from trees in the genus Santalum. When applied to the skin, it protects wounds, sores, boils, and pimples from developing infections or from becoming septic. The essential oil of sandalwood soothes the skin and helps scars and spots to heal much faster. Sandalwood oil relieves the skin from inflammation and irritation, and aids in the cure of infections.

Sea Salt
Sea salt is salt that is produced by the evaporation of seawater. It is used in cosmetics.

Shea Butter
Shea butter, also known as karite butter, is a cream-colored fatty substance made from the nuts of karite nut trees that grow in the savannah regions of West and Central Africa. Shea butter has been

used to help heal burns, sores, scars, dermatitis, psoriasis, dandruff, and stretch marks. It may also help diminish wrinkles by moisturizing the skin, promoting cell renewal, and increasing circulation. Shea butter also contains cinnamic acid, a substance that helps protect the skin from harmful UV rays.

Spearmint Essential Oil

Spearmint essential is made through steam distillation. It is known for its effects on the digestive system, and for relieving aches and pains. Spearmint is loaded with vitamins, antioxidants and vital nutrients

Sunflower Oil

Sunflower oil is the non-volatile oil pressed from the seeds of sunflower. Sunflower oil, rich in vitamin E, is specifically related to improving skin health and regenerating cells. You can see an increased reduction in scars, quicker wound healing, and a healthier natural glow to your skin.

Sweet Almond Oil (*Prunus amygdalus dulcis*)

Sweet almond oil is a pale yellow oil that is derived by pressing the kernels of sweet and bitter almonds. Known for its excellent nourishing abilities, sweet almond oil is commonly found in soaps, massage oils, and other cosmetic products.

Sweet Orange Essential Oil (*Citrus sinensis*)

Sweet Orange oil is extracted as a by-product of orange juice production by centrifugation, producing a cold-pressed oil. Sweet Orange essential oil is known to promote the production of collagen as well as increase the blood flow to the skin. It is helpful at soothing dry, irritated skin as well as acne-prone skin. It is excellent for rubbing on calluses on the feet.

Tangerine Oil

The essential oil of tangerine is extracted by cold compression of its peels. Tangerine oil is known for its antifungal and antiseptic properties, making it a popular ingredient in skin care formulas. It's a great remedy for acne, skin impurities, helps treat dandruff, dry scalp and other scalp infections.

Tapioca Starch

Tapioca is a starch extracted from the cassava plant. Although it can be used as a flour for baking, it's mainly used as a thickener.

Tea Tree Essential Oil *(Melaleuca alternifolia)*

Tea tree oil is extracted by steam distillation of tea tree leaves and twigs. Tea tree oil's powerful disinfectant properties make it effective in treating a variety of cuts, sores, abscesses, and wounds. Acne, oily skin, herpes, warts and cold sores also react well to topical applications of tea tree oil. Tea tree oil works well on a wide range of skin problems, including blemishes, rashes and warts. Effective in fighting acne, tea tree oil also provides an effective treatment for fungal infection of the fingernails, an increasing problem that may be linked to the growing use of artificial fingernails.

Thyme Oil

Thyme (Thymus vulgaris) is an herb that belongs to the mint family (Lamiaceae). It's currently cultivated throughout the world, and the leaves are commonly dried and used as culinary seasoning. Thyme oil is antiseptic, antibacterial, antispasmodic, hypertensive and has calming properties. Thyme oil is one of the strongest antioxidants known. Thyme supports the immune, respiratory, digestive, nervous and other body systems.

Vanilla Essential Oil

The essential oil of vanilla is extracted from fermented vanilla beans. The antioxidant property of vanilla essential oil neutralizes free radicals and protects the body from wear and tear and infections. Vanilla essential oil is an effective antidepressant and mood lifter. This oil has relaxing and calming effects that provide relief from anxiety, anger, and restlessness.

Vegetable Glycerin

Glycerin is a simple polyol compound that is extracted from triglycerides found in different plant and animal sources, which when treated with alcohol give glycerin as a byproduct. Its excellent moisturizing properties aid in keeping skin looking young and healthy as retaining moisture is vital for keeping skin in its best condition. It also draws oxygen into the skin, which is beneficial for anti-aging and effective against dry skin.

Vitamin D Oil

Vitamin D is actually a hormone. Some of the many benefits of Vitamin D for the body include the formation of healthy and strong teeth, bones, and nails.

Vitamin E Oil

Vitamin E is an antioxidant that occurs naturally in foods such as nuts, seeds, and leafy green vegetables. Because of its antioxidant activity, vitamin E is vital to protecting skin cells and fights with elements that produce cell damaging free radicals. Vitamin E also helps reduce the appearance of stretch marks and prevents the appearance of age spots by rejuvenating the skin cells over your body.

Wheat Germ Oil

Wheat germ oil is extracted from the germ of the wheat kernel, which makes up only 2.5% by weight of the kernel. Wheat germ oil is very high in vitamin E and has the highest content of vitamin E of any food that has not undergone prior preparation or vitamin fortification. The Wheat Germ Oil benefits for hair and skin are too amazing to ignore. Wheat germ oil is also rich in vitamins A, B, D, and E, and high in antioxidants — wheat germ is one of the best oils to support collagen production repairing and healing skin conditions.

Wintergreen Essential Oil (*Gaultheria procumbens*)

Wintergreen essential oil is created by steam distilling the leaves of the plant. It soothes discomfort in the muscles and joints and promotes healthy respiratory function.

Ylang Ylang (*Cananga odorata*)

Ylang ylang essential oil comes from flower petals of the large, tropical ylang ylang tree. Ylang ylang means "flower of flowers" Ylang ylang oil benefits any type of skin but is especially effective in treating oily skin because it balances oil production and reduces excessive oiliness. By fighting bacterial infections, it helps control acne and blemishes. Ylang ylang oil softens and soothes skin and stimulates new cell growth. It reportedly can ward off wrinkles and premature aging because it relaxes facial muscles and releases facial tension that can contribute to lines and sagging skin.

ESSENTIAL OIL SAFETY

Do not use essential oils if you are pregnant or planning on becoming pregnant without consulting a doctor. DO not use essential oils on children. ALWAYS consult a doctor before using any essential oil as many of these oils are not recommended for use with many health conditions!

NEVER apply undiluted essential oils to your skin. Always dilute essential oils with a carrier oil before use.

Essential Oils can cause allergic reactions for some people. When using an essential oil topically for the first time make sure to do a small patch test on your skin first. To do this:

Place 1-2 drops of diluted essential oil on your forearm or back. Wrap the area with a bandage to cover. Do not get the area wet. If you feel any irritation or sensitivity – remove the bandage and wash the area immediately with soap and water.

If no irritations occur after 48 hours, the diluted essential oil should be safe to use on your skin. Never apply undiluted essential oils directly to your skin. If sensitivity or irritation develops wash the area immediately with soap and water and stop use.

Many essential oils are phototoxic and cause irritation or blisters when exposed to UVA rays. Do not expose skin that has been treated with phototoxic essential oils to UVA rays for a minimum of 24 hours after use.

ALWAYS CONSULT A PHYSICAN B
EFORE USING
ANY ESSENTIAL OIL

PRESERVATIVES

Every time you put your hands into your cream, your hands always have some sort of bacteria on it. Vitamin E is not a preservative. Should you choose to use a preservative, the following are available. Normally, you do not need a preservative in butters because they do not contain water. Always have clean hands before putting then into your creams.

Germaben ii-Nothing natural. Mixture of poly glycol, paraben, commonly used preservative.

Optifin-Paraben free, formaldehyde free preservative. Not all natural.

Optifin ND-Lighter version of optifin.

When buying butters please buy from recommended resources. Lots of products today are mixed with synthetic things.

HARMFUL INGREDIENTS IN COSMETICS

Last year more than $8 billion was spent on researching health and skin care products in the U.S. Modern testing is proving time and time again that many ingredients used in skin care products aren't good for the body or the skin. When purchasing beauty products, always check out the labels on the container and be sure you know about the hidden hazards and harmful ingredients in them!

It is your responsibility to read the labels on moisturizers and other personal care products. You will most likely find some of the following harmful-carcinogenic ingredients in the products that you are now using!

Propylene Glycol - Called a humectant in cosmetics, it is really "industrial anti-freeze" and the major ingredient in brake and hydraulic fluid.

Mineral Oil (Petrolatum, Petroleum) - Comes from crude oil (petroleum) used in industry as metal cutting fluid. May suffocate the skin by forming an oil film.

Petrolatum, Petroleum, Mineral Oil - Same properties as Mineral Oil. Industrially it is used as a grease component.

Sodium Lauryl Sulfate (SLS) And Sodium Laureth Sulfate (Sles) - Potentially, SLS is perhaps the most harmful ingredient in personal-care products. Industrial uses of SLS include: garage floor cleaners, engine degreasers and car wash soaps.

Lanolin - Lanolin has been found to be a common skin sensitizer causing allergic contact skin rashes. Lanolin usually contains pesticides and dioxins.

Mineral Oil - An oil manufactured from crude oil. The fact that mineral oil does not penetrate the skin well makes it inappropriate for use as an absorption base in a skin cream of any kind. In fact, mineral oil-containing cosmetics can produce symptoms similar to dry skin by inhibiting the natural moisturizing factor of your skin. Petrolatum, paraffin or paraffin oil and propylene glycol are other common cosmetic forms of mineral oil. It also has a tendency to dissolve the skin's own natural oil and thereby increase dehydration.

Propylene Glycol - found in most moisturizers, is industrial anti-freeze. Your skin needs water, not anti-freeze. According to the Material Safety Data Sheets, Propylene glycol can penetrate the skin and cause liver abnormalities and kidney damage.

Centers for Disease control: http://www.cdc.gov/

RECOMMENDED SUPPLIERS

Mountain Rose Herbs (https://www.mountainroseherbs.com)

From Nature with Love (www.fromnaturewithlove.com)

Soapers Choice (https://www.soaperschoice.com)

Amazon (http://www.amazon.com)

Bulk Apothecary (www.bulkapothecary.com)

Brambleberry (https://www.brambleberry.com)

Whole Foods (local market)

NowFoods.com (https://www.nowfoods.com)

Aura Cacia (https://www.auracacia.com)

RECOMMENDED UTENSILS

You will need the following utensils to get you started.

- Pyrex measuring cup – 1, 2 and 4 cups. You will use these to heat your butters in a microwave and can also use it as a mixing bowl.
- Good stainless steel knife - for cutting butters.
- Stainless steel spoon or utensils – Stainless steel utensils can be completely sanitized and can be used again and again.
- Stainless steel measuring cups – perfect for multiple use and well made.
- Stick blender – fits well in a Pyrex cup to blend your butters.
- Hand mixer – to mix large amounts of butters.
- Double Boiler – to heat your butters and waxes.
- Wooden spoons or skewers - for stirring. Some metals may chemically react to some essential oils.
- Grater – For grating beeswax and cocoa butter into small pieces for quicker melting.
- Air tight containers – Whether the products are for personal use or as gifts, you can package your body butters in mason jars, decorative jars or vessels sold especially for these kinds of products. Whichever container you use, make sure it has an airtight lid.

Sanitizing Utensils Prior to Use

34

Have on hand, 90% rubbing alcohol in a spray bottle.

Wash your utensils and bowl first by hand or in the dishwasher.

Dry with a clean towel or paper towel.

Spray everything down with alcohol.

Wipe each utensil with a paper towel.

Spray again.

Let air dry

HERE'S TO HEALTHY BEAUTIFUL SKIN

The skin is a living breathing organ that requires all the nutrients that other organs need to stay healthy. The exposed layer of skin is called the epidermis and is most vulnerable to environmental damage.

Maintain Beautiful Healthy Skin

- Stay hydrated – drink plenty of water.
- Keep skin clean - Cleansing is the most basic element of any skin care routine as it removes excess dirt, pollutants and pore-clogging oil from the epidermis to remain blemish free.
- Use a sunscreen to help protect your skin from diseases like skin cancer and help prevent the signs of skin aging that comes from the exposure to sun.
- Stay away from cleansers that contain harsh chemicals and fragrances that may strip the skin of essential oils and leave behind a drying residue that may irritate sensitive skin.
- Use a moisturizer daily for protection from the sun.
- Whatever soap you use may be absorbed into your bloodstream through your skin. Always use natural, chemical-free soap.

What You Should Use on Your Skin

- Authentic African Black soap or any other natural soap that does not include any harmful chemicals.
- Shea butter
- Water
- Natural products
- Chemical free products.

Fragrance free products

As skin is a living, breathing organ, it makes absolutely no sense to slap synthetic skincare products on it. Never put harsh cleansers or chemicals on your skin. Remember your moto, if you can't eat it yourself, don't feed it to your skin.

Read the labels on your current products.

I encourage you to check out the labels on your hair, skin, body, dental, personal hygiene, and beauty cosmetics. Be sure you know about the hidden carcinogens and harmful ingredients in them! If there are harmful ingredients in them it's time for a change.

NICE & NATURAL HAIR

Your hair is your crowning glory, own it, love it, enjoy it.

Your hair is your crowning glory it's just a pity that what we put into it can leave it dry and dull and even brittle. Here are some effective hair remedies that will infuse some much needed bounce and shine back into dull and lifeless hair.

Not only is your hair your crowning glory, but hair serves several other functions as well;

- it protects the scalp against the harmful effects of sun exposure,

- facilitates sweat evaporation,

- helps control body heat and

- blocks dirt and dust.

Prevent Damaged Hair

Hair can become damaged by overuse of hair dryers, hair straighteners, curling irons, or by harsh chemicals like those found in hair dye and hair straightening solutions. To help alleviate damage, rehydrate your hair with a homemade shea butter hair conditioner which works deeply to penetrate your roots and replenish each hair shaft with necessary vitamins and nutrients.

Shea butter is a natural moisturizer that can fortify and add shine to your hair. By using shea butter in your hair care routine, you can give it radiant shine and bring your hair back to life. With a few tips and recipes, you can discover the best way to use shea butter in your hair.

They say that a woman's hair is her crowning glory. Even so, all women have those days when we wish we could cover every unwieldy strand! Here are a few more tips and recipes to help you maintain that mane.

- Get a good haircut! It all begins right here. Without a good haircut, nothing else you do will give you the results you want.

- If you absolutely must trim your hair at home, do it right! Purchase a pair of professional hair cutting scissors and use them for nothing else. Not to cut out pictures for the kid's class project, not to trim a frayed edge from a piece of clothing. Use them for cutting hair . . . period! Take care of them properly and they will last you for years to come.

- Keep your hair clean! There's nothing worse than dirty, oily hair that hangs in clumps.

- Use a natural chemical-free shampoo for your hair type. Not all hair is created equal.

Natural Hair Growth Cream

Ingredients:
4 tablespoons of shea butter
2 tablespoons of coconut oil
1/2 cup of aloe vera gel
1 tablespoon jojoba oil
1 tablespoon castor oil
Method: in a double boiler (or microwave), melt shea butter and coconut oil. After melting, add jojoba oil and castor oil. Allow to cool for about 5 minutes, then add aloe vera gel. Whip together with hand mixer into a cream consistency. Scoop into a clean container.

Basic Natural Hair Conditioner

Ingredients:

1 teaspoon shea butter

1 teaspoon vegetable glycerin

1 tablespoon beeswax

1/2 teaspoon vitamin E (or 2 capsules)

1/2 cup distilled water

5 drops grapefruit seed extract

5 drops lavender essential oil

Method: Melt the beeswax carefully in a double boiler, when it starts melting, put it away from the heat, the rest will melt on its own. When the wax is liquid, add shea butter and glycerin. Shea butter does not stand heat very good, so be a little careful here. In a separate pot on the stove or in the microwave, gently warm the water just until lukewarm. Do NOT skip this step or your conditioner will separate later. Slowly pour the water into the oil mixture, stirring constantly with a wire whisk until the mixture is creamy and smooth. Let the mixture cool a little so the essential oils don't evaporate too quickly when you add them. Stir in the lavender essential oil, vitamin E and the grapefruit seed extract. Pour the natural hair conditioner into a clean, sterilized dark glass or PET plastic bottle and allow it to cool before putting the lid on. Don't worry if it doesn't thicken immediately - it thickens as it cools down to room temperature. Shake the bottle occasionally as the conditioner cools to prevent the ingredients from separating. Store in a cool, dark place.

Shea Butter Conditioner

The simplest and most effective homemade hair conditioner for damaged hair uses only shea butter, a rich substance that coats hair strands and locks in moisture. To begin: wet hair as normal, then massage two to three tablespoons of shea butter into hair. Thoroughly massage scalp and coat the tips of hair strands. If hair is not thoroughly coated, work in an additional tablespoon. Allow to sit for 10 to 15 minutes. Once time has elapsed, rinse hair out as normal and wash using natural chemical-free shampoo. While hair is still wet, comb strands slowly and carefully using a wide-tooth comb if necessary, to discourage split ends. Allow hair to air dry or secure in a loose ponytail. If possible, avoid harsh tools, such as hair dryers, curling irons and hair straighteners, and minimize hair product use that contain harmful chemicals. It's very essential to have hair trimmed every one to two months to remove split ends and promote healthy, strong hair. Shea butter conditioner can be reapplied once every month to promote healthy hair growth. Shea butter is rich in vitamins and can be beneficial when used on your scalp and hair because it also moisturizes. Olive oil can be combined with shea butter to create a homemade scalp and hair treatment. Olive oil is not only a great deep conditioner, but it also can control dandruff.

Shea Butter Hair Conditioner #1

This is one of the recipes that work excellently as a hair conditioner.

Ingredients:
1 tablespoon shea butter
1 tablespoon regular store-bought hair conditioner
½ tablespoon extra virgin olive oil
Few drops essential oil (according to preference)
Method: Let the shea butter soften at room temperature. Let it not melt. Now add all the other ingredients into the shea butter and stir vigorously. Pour the mixture into a bottle or any container that can be closed tightly.

Shea Butter Conditioner Recipe #2

This recipe helps seal moisture into the hair and provides hold for hairstyles.
Ingredients:
3/4 cup shea butter
2 teaspoons extra virgin coconut oil
1 teaspoons of extra virgin olive oil
3 teaspoons aloe vera gel
A few drops of vanilla fragrance oil (optional)
Method: Make sure the shea butter is softened to room temperature. Melt the coconut oil into liquid using a double boiler. Mix in your olive oil. Mix in a teaspoon of aloe vera gel. Use this conditioner after moisturizing your hair with your favorite water-based moisturizer, or just plain water. This mix should not be used on its own as it doesn't provide any moisture and will prevent your hair from absorbing any moisture, leaving your hair dry. The shea

butter helps to seal in moisture and the oils help to further seal and give your hair shine. The aloe vera gel provides hold, making it great for holding styles like twists, naturals, and twist-outs!

Olive Oil Hair and Scalp Conditioner

Ingredients:

1 tablespoon of softened shea butter

1/2 tablespoon of extra virgin olive oil

Method: Add the olive oil to the shea butter and mix the two ingredients together. Massage the homemade olive oil conditioner hair and scalp remedy into your scalp and using a wide tooth comb, run some of it through your hair. You can let it sit overnight and wash it out in the morning or wear it as a leave-in conditioner. You can add a few drops of coconut essential oil to the mixture to create a pleasant scent.

Shea Butter Hair Whip

Ingredients:

9 ounces shea butter

½ cup coconut oil

2 tablespoons extra virgin olive oil

Method: Whip softened shea butter, coconut oil and extra virgin olive oil together with mixer for 20 minutes. Add your choice of fragrance and whip for 20 more minutes. Apply when hair is damp. For maximum results, use shea butter hair whip in your hair twice a week.

Shea Butter Recipe for Extra Dry Hair

Ingredients:

2 tablespoons shea butter

2 tablespoons castor oil

Method: Blend shea butter and castor oil together and apply to hair. Comb through with a large tooth comb.

TIP: A great rejuvenator: Have someone give you a scalp massage.

Shea Bee Hair Pomade
Ingredients:
2 ounces (jojoba oil or almond oil)
1 ounce beeswax
1.5 ounces shea butter
¼ ounces essential oil (peppermint, rosemary, lavender or a combination of all three)
Method: Melt the beeswax carefully in a double boiler, when it starts melting, remove it from the heat, the rest will melt on its own. When the wax is liquid, add shea butter and jojoba or almond oil. Let cool, then add the essential oil(s). If your hair doesn't like the wax, use it for your lips, it's a good way to use up the wax.

Heavy Hold Hair Styling Pomade
Ingredients:
¾ cup beeswax pastilles
½ cup unrefined shea butter
½ cup jojoba oil
1 teaspoon vitamin E (optional)
2 tablespoon arrowroot powder (optional)
Method: Melt the beeswax carefully in a double boiler, when it starts melting, remove it from the heat, the rest will melt on its own. When the wax is liquid, add shea butter and oil. Let cool, then add arrowroot powder.

Medium Hold Hair Styling Pomade
Ingredients:
¾ cup unrefined shea butter
½ cup beeswax pastilles
½ cup jojoba oil
1 teaspoon vitamin E
2 tablespoons arrowroot powder (optional)
30 drops rosemary essential oil or part rosemary essential oil
20 drops lime essential oil or part lime essential oil
10 drops vanilla absolute or part vanilla absolute
Method: In a double boiler or a pyrex bowl in a saucepan of boiling water melt the beeswax and shea butter, stirring every so often. Mix together arrowroot powder, jojoba oil, and essential oils

in a small bowl. Using a fork, stir until the arrowroot is dissolved into the oil. If using Vitamin E to lengthen the shelf life of the pomade, poke the vitamin E pills squeezing the contents into the bowl and let cool until hardened. When the beeswax shea mixture is melted, remove it from the heat and add arrowroot/jojoba oil/essential oil mixture. Using your hand mixer, blend the hair pomade until it begins to turn into a pudding-like texture. Scoop into your designated container and store in a cool dark place. The pomade will harden further overnight. Use only a small pea sized amount on hair. A little goes a long way!

Shea Butter Hair Cream

Ingredients:
4 tablespoons shea butter
2 tablespoons cocoa butter
4 tablespoons extra virgin olive oil
few drops ylang ylang essential oil
Method: In a double boiler or microwave, melt the shea butter and cocoa butter. Pour the melted butters into a mixing bowl. Next add the extra virgin olive oil to the melted butters. Add the ylang ylang essential oil for fragrance. Place the mixture over another bowl filled with ice. This will allow the mixture you have prepared to cool properly and set. Whisk it thoroughly and place it into a container.

Shea Butter Pretreatment

This hair cream recipe is a very good moisturizer and works especially well on hair that has undergone chemical treatments or has been relaxed.

Ingredients:
1 teaspoon shea butter
1 teaspoon extra virgin olive oil or grapeseed oil
2 drops lavender oil
2 drops rosemary oil
1 drop tea tree oil
Method: Mix all the ingredients together and comb through hair. Cover with a plastic cap. Shampoo 20 minutes later.

Invest in your hair, it is the crown

you never take off

FABULOUS FACE

**"I'm a firm believer that if you focus on
good skin care, you really won't need a
lot of makeup."
Demi Moore**

The skin on your face is thinner than the skin on your body, except for the chest, and deserves a bit more TLC.

For as long as one can remember, it has always been the pursuit of many to keep their youthful looks, even at great costs. And currently, the trend has not changed. Now more than ever, methods, techniques and treatments meant to retain that youthful glow flourish everywhere. Anti-ageing goods and services account for billions of dollars spent in the hopes of delaying the onset of skin ageing. Unfortunately, many have been misinformed on how and why the skin ages - misleading these same people into buying products that only offer short-lived, if not unsuccessful and disappointing, results.

Areas of the face that are dry should be gently cleansed, preferably with cold creams containing shea butter and washed with lukewarm water then pat dry with a towel without rubbing.

Oily parts should be thoroughly cleansed and kept dry to avoid breakouts of acne. Oily areas are so sensitive that any incorrect application of medications and creams may cause acne and other irritations to erupt.

The skin consists of microscopically small, flat scales that constantly flake off, thereby revealing the new skin beneath the outer, older layer of scales. In millions of people the old, tired, dead, dry outer scales do not peel off promptly, slowing new growth and leaving their skin dry, ashen, dull and lifeless. This is known as the "old age look". You should exfoliate dead skin cells every week with an inexpensive gentle face puff. Your skin will look more youthful and will shine with a joyous new life.

Mother Nature's Wonder Cream

Create your own facial cream. Here are a few excellent creams that you can create with natural ingredients right from Mother Nature:

FrankinShea Face Cream
Ingredients:
2 tablespoons shea butter
2 drops rose essential oil
4 drops frankincense essential oil
Method: Let your shea butter soften at room temperature. Mix it by hand. No need to mix it with electric mixer. Mix all ingredients together and apply after washing your face. Leave on for 30 minutes, and then wipe off with tissue.

FrankinShea Cocoa Almond Cream
Ingredients:
1/2 cup cocoa butter
1/2 cup Shea butter
2 tablespoons jojoba oil
2 tablespoons sweet almond oil
40 drops frankincense essential oil
Method: In a double boiler or microwave, melt the cocoa butter. Combine melted cocoa butter, shea butter, jojoba oil, and sweet almond oil in a bowl. Once it is cooled, use your electric mixer to whip it up. Whip until nice and fluffy, then add in the frankincense and whip until combined.

Nature's Best Wrinkle Smoother

Unlike Cleopatra, we now live in the nuclear age and wrinkles can become a thing of the past. The best cure for wrinkles is to never have them in the first place! If you are like most of us, you didn't listen to your Mom when she tried to tell you to stop squinting! Shea butter is nature's best wrinkle smoother. Massage your face with pure shea butter at least three times a week and you will see nature's wonder butter at work.

Nature's Wrinkle-Reducing Face Cream
Ingredients:
1/4 cup shea butter
1/4 cup organic coconut oil
8-10 drops frankincense essential oil
5-7 drops lavender essential oil
Method: Using a double boiler or microwave, melt the shea butter and coconut oil together until liquid. Do not over heat. Remove from heat and let cool for about 30 minutes. Drop in frankincense and lavender essential oils and stir. Wait for mix to partially solidify (if necessary, place in refrigerator for a few minutes). Then whip with your hand mixer until you achieve a butter-like consistency (few minutes). Store in a 4 oz. jar. This should keep for 6-12 months in your bathroom cupboard.

Always use Organic Natural Shea Butter

Stop stressing!

Easier said than done? All that stress that you keep bottled up inside creates those worry lines and wrinkles.

Beautiful Eyes

Use shea butter as a special under-the-eye moisturizer to keep tissue around the eyes soft and pliable. The skin around the eyes is very thin and easily damaged. Before bed, dab a little shea/grapeseed butter around the eyes and wipe off with tissue.

Shea/Grapeseed Butter Eye Cream

Ingredients:
4 tablespoons shea butter
1 teaspoon grapeseed oil

Method: Whip together by hand until creamy. Store in a nice clean jar.

Luscious Lips

Don't forget Shea butter for your lips. They want to be healthy too!

This is a fabulous recipe for natural lip butter. It will help keep your lips soft and supple in the winter season.

Luscious Lip Balm
This lip balm recipe is very effective for dry and cracked lips.
Ingredients:
1 teaspoon beeswax
1 teaspoon extra virgin olive oil
1/2 teaspoon castor oil
1 teaspoon shea butter
Method: First melt beeswax in the top of a double boiler. Add shea butter and stir it by hand. When shea butter is melted and blended with beeswax remove it from the heat. Add olive oil and castor oil drop by drop while mixing it. Carefully pour into lip balm tubes or pots. Allow to cool for about 20 minutes before using. Enjoy!!

The castor oil will give it a nice shine, and the shea butter and beeswax are good conditioners.

Natural Makeup Remover

Use pure shea butter for removing makeup.

Natural Face Mask

Clay Face Mask for Oily Skin
Ingredients:
1 tablespoon European clay
1 tablespoon shea butter

1 teaspoon distilled water

Clay face mask for dry skin
1 tablespoon European clay
1 tablespoon shea butter
1 teaspoon distilled water
5 drops of jojoba oil
5 drops of lavender oil

Method: Make sure shea butter is room temperature soft. Mix together with European clay. Thoroughly cover the face and neck avoiding sensitive areas and the eyes, allow to set for 15-20 minutes, rinse off and apply moisturizer.

Natural Acne Relief

Non-greasy Acne Cream
Great for acne and dark spots
Ingredients:
5 drops lavender
5 drops geranium
5 drops bergamot
2 tablespoons shea butter

Method: While shea butter is soft, hand mix all ingredients together. Massage face nightly with acne cream until face is clear of acne and dark spots. Always wipe off with clean tissue before washing your face.

Bottom Line

Now you see, you do not have to break the bank to have soft baby smooth facial skin that glows. Yet, in trying not to be too cheap we must start to go back to our roots in the natural. Everywhere you turn there is talk about anti-aging and healing remedies on the internet, television and even in casual work conversations. So many overhyped products promising remedies fly off the beauty store shelves daily but the truth is, the answer to perfect skin lies in mother nature's gift - the authentic shea butter. Bottom line; pamper your face with Mother Nature.

"Every woman should learn how to be

her own skincare expert."
Bobbi Brown

Ear Lobes

Often, we may buy pretty but cheap earrings. This may sometimes lead to sore ear lobes. To remedy this, try this recipe.

Ingredients:
1 tablespoon shea butter
2 drops tea tree oil
Method: Mix together well. Take a small amount and with your thumb and forefinger massage it onto the front and back of the ear lobe. Also put a small amount onto the earring posts before inserting into pierced ear holes.

Nice Neck

Shea Butter and Aloe Vera Neck Cream
Ingredients:
4 tablespoons shea butter
3 teaspoons aloe vera gel
2 teaspoons rose water
1 teaspoon argan oil
5 to 7 drops of rose essential oil
½ teaspoon or 1 capsule of vitamin E oil (optional)
Method: Scoop out the shea butter and place it in a medium sized mixing bowl. If your shea butter is hard, soften it using a double boiler or microwave. Whip it with a hand mixer for a minute till its smooth and fluffy. Add the aloe vera gel and whip again till mixed. While whipping, slowly add the rose water little by little until fully incorporated. Finally, add the argan oil, vitamin E oil, rose essential oil and blend the mixture into a soft cream for about 7-10 minutes, then place it in the refrigerator for 15 minutes then take it out and whip again for 10 minutes. Your whipped shea butter and aloe vera cream is ready! Spoon it into a sterilized clean jar, and store in a clean dry place.

Apply liberally on your face, neck, hands and whole body. You can also use it to seal moisture into your beautiful hair!

BODY BEAUTIFUL

"Invest in your skin, it's going to be with you for a long time."
Linden Tyler

True beauty begins from the inside out. Don't you wish there was some way to wriggle your nose and regain that soft skin you had as a child? Well, until someone comes up with the true Fountain of Youth, we are stuck with what we have.

The best route to healthy skin is to take care of what you have now. Sounds simple, doesn't it? The truth is that your skin takes a beating from the environment every single day. Here are some of our favorite tips for keeping your skin fresh and healthy:

- Stay hydrated, and drink plenty of water! That doesn't mean soda, or caffeine or any other type of liquid even if it is low cal. You need fluid that will hydrate and flush your body free of toxins. Make sure you are drinking at least 6-8 glasses a day!

- Protect your skin from harmful ultra violet (UV) rays. We all love the sun. We love being in it and we love having a beautiful tan. The truth is you can poison yourself with too much sunshine. UV rays cause skin cancer, and if that isn't bad enough, it causes your skin to age faster than it should, contributing to unsightly wrinkles. If you must play in the sun, make certain you are using an adequate sun screen. Don't leave home without it!

- Apply your sun screen even if you only make a quick trip to the grocery store. Yes, you can get harmful UV rays even while driving your car!

- The first daily must is the most obvious: Healthy skin must be clean.

Here are a few recipes crafted with a blend of plant-derived oils combined with shea butter that will nourish your skin and provide a smooth silky glide during massage. Create your at-home beauty treatment that stabilizes the senses, nourishes the body and comforts the spirit.

Balms

Balms are fragrant preparations used to heal or soothe the skin.

Coconut Cream Balm
This balm will sooth dry skin
Ingredients:
3 tablespoons coconut oil
4 tablespoons shea butter
1 tablespoon cocoa butter
40 drops vanilla or sweet orange essential oil
Method: In double boiler or microwave, warm coconut, shea and cocoa butter until melted. Remove from heat and let cool for 15 minutes. Add essential oils and stir.

Lotion Bars

A lotion bar is a solid moisturizer. It bears resemblance to a soap bar, but it functions as a lotion. Usually made from natural ingredients, lotion bars stay solid as long as they are kept at room temperature or lower. They're activated by body heat and can be used anywhere on the body.

Golden Oasis Lotion Bar
Ingredients:
6 ounces cocoa butter
5 ounces shea butter
5 ounces aloe vera gel
.5 ounce palm oil
.5 ounce wheat germ oil
.5 ounce sweet almond oil
2 vitamin E capsules (emptied)
Few drops of your favorite essential oil

Method: In a double boiler, melt the cocoa butter, shea butter. Remove from heat and add the aloe vera gel, palm oil, wheat germ oil, vitamin E, favorite essential oil, and sweet almond oil. Stir gently and put into a mold or container and refrigerate. You can replace the palm oil and sweet almond oil with other oils, depending on what you have on hand, and the lotion bar still works great.

Sunset Butter Lotion Bar
Ingredients:
3 ounces beeswax
3 ounces cocoa butter
3 ounces shea butter
3 ounces jojoba or any other liquid oil such as olive oil
Method: First you need to melt beeswax, cocoa butter and shea butter in a double boiler. Once it's all melted you can stir in the liquid oil, if you want, you can also add a little fragrance or essential oil to make some nice perfumed bars. Pour the melted oils into container then allow to cool and harden. Gently remove the hardened bars from their molds and your home-made solid body butter bars are now ready for use.

Just Butter Lotion Bar
Ingredients:
2 ounces cocoa butter
2 ounces beeswax
2 ounces shea butter
Method: Melt all ingredients together in the top of a double boiler and pour into a container or mold. Be sure to mix ingredients well.

Cocoa/Shea Butter Lotion Bars
Ingredients:
1-part beeswax
1-part cocoa butter
1-part shea butter
1-part coconut oil
Method: Melt all ingredients together and pour into a container or mold.

Avocado Bee Lotion Bar
Ingredients:

Greasy at first but absorbs right into the skin
1/3 Beeswax
1/3 Olive Oil
1/3 split evenly between Avocado Oil and Shea Butter
 Method: Melt the wax and oils in a double boiler, add essential oils if you wish and pour into whatever small mold you like. Allow to harden.

Lavender Lotion Bar

Ingredients:
1/2 cup oil (sunflower; olive; almond etc.)
1/2 cup beeswax
1/2 cup shea butter
10-15 drops Lavender essential oil
Method: In a double boiler, melt oil, beeswax and shea butter together. Remove from heat and add lavender oil. To make it harder add more beeswax; to make it softer, add more oil. Pour into a container or mold and refrigerate. Store in an air tight container, away from the sunlight or in the refrigerator.

Coconut Oil Lotion Bar

Ingredients:
½ cup beeswax
½ cup coconut oil
½ cup grapeseed oil, apricot oil or sweet almond
½ cup shea butter
1 teaspoon of your favorite essential oil
Method: Melt all together in a double boiler or microwave and pour into a container or mold.

Earthy and Sweet Lotion Bar

This simple homemade lotion bar combines the wonderful aromas of cocoa butter, lime, lavender and patchouli in a skin soothing oil blend that will leave you feeling silky smooth.

Ingredients:
1/2 cup beeswax
1/4 cup cocoa butter
1/4 cup shea butter

2 tablespoons castor oil
2 tablespoons macadamia oil
1/4 cup coconut oil
1/2 teaspoon lavender essential oil
1/2 teaspoon patchouli essential oil
1/2 teaspoon lime essential oil
1 teaspoon vitamin E oil
Method: Prepare a styrofoam mold or lined cupcake pan. In a double boiler, melt beeswax, shea butter and cocoa butter together over medium heat.   As the mixture is melting, add the castor, coconut and macadamia oils. Once the heated mixture is completely liquid, remove from heat and add the essential oils plus E. Whisk together for 15 to 20 seconds to evenly disperse the essential oils and pour into your styrofoam mold or lined cupcake pan. If you fill each cup ¾ of the way full, you will end up with 6 lotion bars. Let cool before removing from pan. Use it to cleanse oily skin or combine with eucalyptus for a purifying circulation.

Every Day Lotion Bar
Ingredients:
1/3 beeswax
1/3 olive oil
1/3 shea butter
Method: Melt the wax and oils in a double boiler, scent if you wish and pour into whatever small mold you like. Allow to harden. Greasy at first but absorbs right into the skin.

Lavender Vanilla Avocado Lotion Bar
For a nourishing and skin softening homemade lotion bar, try this rich combination of avocado oil, cocoa butter, coconut oil, lavender and vanilla essential oils. This bar does not include shea butter.

Ingredients
1/4 cup beeswax beads or grated beeswax
1/4 cup cocoa butter, chopped or grated
1/4 cup coconut oil
2 tablespoons avocado oil
24 drops Vanilla Precious Essentials
24 drops lavender essential oil
Method: In a double boiler, heat the beeswax and cocoa butter

until melted. Stir until the solids are completely liquid. Add the coconut oil and avocado oil and mix well. Remove from heat and add the essential oils, then give the blend a final stir. Pour into muffin tins lined with paper baking cups – or for one large bar, a small loaf pan. Place in the refrigerator (or freezer) until set. Makes 2 muffin cup-sized bars.

Lovable Blend Lotion Bar
Ingredients:
1 cup coconut oil
1 cup shea butter
(can substitute for cocoa butter or do ½ & ½ if preferred)
1 cup beeswax
1 teaspoon vitamin E oil
25-50 drops (total) of the following oils:
Naturally Loveable Oil Blend (Nowfoods.com)
Lavender oil
Rose absolute oil
Jasmine absolute oil
Vanilla essential oil
Method: Melt everything EXCEPT essential oils in double boiler while stirring constantly until completely melted. Have essential oil ready to go since the mixture will harden quickly. Turn heat to the lowest possible setting and add oils and stir. Pour the mixture into the mold of your choice (silicone baking molds are a great option, or you can use cupcake liners in a regular cupcake tin as well). Allow filled molds to cool and harden until they can be popped out of the mold. Use as a moisturizing bar on the body.

No Cocoa Butter Lotion Bar
Ingredients:
1 parts coconut oil
1 part shea butter
1 part beeswax
1-1/2 parts sweet almond oil
Method: Melt all ingredients together in a double boiler and pour into a container or mold. Be sure to mix ingredients well.

All Butter Lotion Bars
Ingredients:
2 ounces cocoa butter
2 ounces beeswax
2 ounces shea butter
Method: Melt all together and pour into a container or mold. Be sure to mix ingredients well. Store in an air tight container, away from the sunlight or in the refrigerator.

Cocoa/Shea Butter Lotion Bars
Ingredients:
1 ounce beeswax
1 ounce cocoa butter
1 ounce shea butter
1 ounce coconut oil
Method: Melt all in a double boiler and pour into a clean container.

Luxurious Lotion Bars
Ingredients:
1 cup of coconut oil
1 cup of shea butter
1 cup of beeswax
1 teaspoon of vitamin E oil
25-50 drops of an essential oil (or blend of favorite oils to your liking)
Method: In a double boiler or microwave, melt all ingredients except essential oils. Stir constantly until completely melted. The mixture will harden quickly so have essential oils prepared and ready to go. Stir and pour into the mold of your choice.

Beautiful Body Butters

Aloe Vera Butter
Ingredients:
6 ounces cocoa butter
5 ounces shea butter
5 ounces aloe vera gel
.5 ounce palm oil
.5 ounce wheat germ oil
.5 ounce sweet almond oil
2 vitamin E capsules (emptied)
5 drops essential oil of choice
Method: Melt the cocoa butter and shea butter together in a double boiler or microwave. Add rest of ingredients and stir until completely combined. Put container in refrigerator until it's almost hardened. Remove from refrigerator and whip with hand mixer until creamy like whipped cream.

Shea Butter for Daily Use
Ingredients:
3 tablespoons unrefined shea butter
1 tablespoon coconut oil
1 tablespoon castor oil
1 tablespoon extra virgin olive oil
Method: Make sure unrefined shea butter and coconut oil are softened at room temperature before you start. Mash them with a fork and add oils. Mash it again a little bit. Mix it with a hand mixer for few minutes and you are done!

Eucalyptus Mint Body Butter
Ingredients:
½ cup coconut oil
6 tablespoons shea butter
6 tablespoons cocoa butter
1 tablespoon olive oil
1-1/2 tablespoon castor oil
10 drops eucalyptus essential oil
3 drops peppermint essential oil

Method: In double boiler, melt coconut oil, shea butter and cocoa butter. Transfer the mixture from double boiler to a glass bowl. Add olive oil, castor oil, eucalyptus oil and peppermint oil and mix well. Refrigerate until mixture is semi-solid then mix with an electric blender until smooth and fluffy. Store in an air tight container, away from the sunlight or in the refrigerator.

Tropical Body Butter

2 tablespoons shea butter
½ tablespoon coconut oil
5 drops lavender oil
5 drops sweet orange oil

Method: Let shea butter and coconut oil soften at room temperature. Mix together by hand. Add essential oils and put in clean container. Or, in double boiler, melt coconut oil and shea butter. Transfer the mixture from double boiler to a glass bowl. Add lavender oil and sweet orange oil and mix well. Refrigerate until mixture is semi-solid then mix with an electric blender until smooth and fluffy. Store in an air tight container, away from the sunlight or in the refrigerator.

Lavender Love body butter

Ingredients:
15 drops progest E
4 teaspoons shea butter
3 ounces coconut oil
7 drops lavender oil
5 drops frankincense essential oil

Method: In double boiler melt shea butter and coconut oil. Transfer to a glass bowl. Add the Progest E, lavender and frankincense essential oil. Mix with spatula until smooth. Leave in refrigerator until it's semi-hard. Remove from refrigerator and whip with mixer until it has the consistency of whipped cream. Store in an airtight container, away from the sunlight or in the refrigerator.

Absolutely Divine Jasmine Body Butter

Here's a great body treatment to give your skin a healthy, nourishing glow. Jasmine is exotic and sensual.

Ingredients:

5 drops Jasmine essential oil
35 drops orange essential oil
1/2 cup coconut oil
1/2 cup shea butter
1 tablespoon jojoba oil
Method: Using a table fork, cream together coconut, shea and jojoba oils. Add Jasmine and orange oil and blend some more. Apply as a skin massage over entire body, (except the face) paying close attention to problem skin areas. Great as an after bath or shower moisturizer.

Aromatic jasmine and olive oil body butter
Ingredients:
1-1/2 cup shea butter
2/3 cup extra virgin olive oil
5 drops jasmine essential oil
Method: In a double boiler, melt shea butter. Add extra virgin olive oil. Transfer to a glass bowl. Let cool for 20 minutes. Add jasmine essential oil. With an electric hand mixer, mix until soft and smooth. Store in an air tight container, away from the sunlight or in the refrigerator.

Chocolate mint whipped body butter
Ingredients:
½ cup cocoa butter
½ cut shea butter
½ cup coconut oil
½ cup jojoba oil
1-2 teaspoons peppermint oil
2 tablespoons cocoa powder
2 teaspoons vitamin D
Method: In a double boiler melt coconut oil, cocoa butter and shea butter. Transfer to a glass bowl. In a separate bowl, mix together jojoba oil with cocoa powder. Add mixture to butters and mix well. Leave at room temperature 45 minutes. Add jojoba and peppermint essential oils and whisk until creamy. Store in an air tight container, away from the sunlight or in the refrigerator.

Coconut Body Butter

Ingredients:

2 tablespoons shea butter

½ tablespoon coconut oil

5 drops lavender oil

5 drops sweet orange oil

Method: Let shea butter and coconut oil soften at room temperature. Mix together by hand. Add essential oils and put in clean container. Or, in a double boiler, melt coconut oil, and shea butter. Transfer the mixture from double boiler to a glass bowl. Add lavender and sweet orange oils and mix well. Refrigerate until mixture is semi-solid then mix with an electric blender until smooth and fluffy. Store in an air tight container, away from the sunlight or in the refrigerator.

Sweet Almond Body Butter

Ingredients:

1 cup shea butter

½ cup coconut oil

½ cup sweet almond oil

Method: Melt shea and coconut oil in double boiler or microwave. Remove from heat. Let cool for 30 minutes. Stir in sweet almond oil. When oil starts to solidify, whip into butter like consistency.

Whipped Vitamin E Body Butter

Ingredients:

1⅓ cups shea butter

½ cup extra virgin olive oil

1 teaspoon vitamin E oil

few drops lavender oil

Method: Put the shea butter in the top of a double boiler or microwave and melt it until it is liquid-like in consistency. Now add the extra virgin olive oil and then put the mixture in refrigerator for at least 40 minutes. Do not let it become completely solid. Now add in vitamin E oil and the lavender essential oil. Take a hand mixer and whip the mixture till the texture of the mixture becomes soft and mousse like. Once you have blended it to achieve the required consistency, scoop this whipped shea butter body butter into containers and use it as and when you want.

Cedarwood and coconut body butter

Cedarwood oil has a warm, woodsy aroma that creates a comforting, uplifting experience.

Ingredients:
1-1/2 cups shea butter
½ cup coconut oil
5 drops cedarwood essential oil
Method: In double boiler melt shea butter and coconut oil. Transfer into a glass bowl. refrigerate for 20 minutes or until partially solid. Do not let it get completely hard. Add cedarwood essential oil. Using a hand mixer, whip until it's soft and smooth. Store in an air tight container, away from the sunlight or in the refrigerator.

Bronze whipped body butter

Ingredients:
1 cup shea butter
½ cup coconut oil
½ cup olive oil
1-2 tablespoon cocoa powder
1 tablespoon ground nutmeg
2 tablespoons ground cinnamon
1 teaspoon vitamin E
5-10 drops essential oil of your choice
Method: In double boiler melt shea and coconut oil. Put into a glass bowl. Add olive oil, cocoa powder, cinnamon, nutmeg, vitamin E and essential oil. Mix well. Refrigerate for 30 minutes until semi solid. Whip with electric mixer until smooth and creamy. Store in an air tight container, away from the sunlight or in the refrigerator.

Evening Primrose Body Cream

This is a shea butter and cocoa butter recipe with geranium oil for cream that is a very good moisturizer and could be helpful for dehydrated or sun damaged skin, and eczema.

Ingredients:
4 teaspoons shea butter

2 teaspoons cocoa butter
1 teaspoon extra virgin grape seed oil
1 teaspoon avocado oil
20 drops Evening Primrose oil
15 drops geranium oil
Method: Melt shea butter and cocoa butters using a double boiler or microwave. Remove it out from the heat and let it cool down to room temperature. Add grapeseed, avocado, evening primrose, and geranium oils. Mix it with a mixer for 5 minutes. Put it in the refrigerator (not in the freezer) for few minutes and mix it again. Don't leave it in the refrigerator for a long time, because it will be too hard for mixing. Put it in a clean jar and let it cool down to room temperature. This cream will have a very nice scent due to Cocoa butter and Geranium oil.

Gorgeous Glow Body Butter
Ingredients:
2 cups organic coconut oil
7 ounces shea butter
1 drop tea tree oil
10-15 drops favorite essential oil
Method: In double boiler melt coconut oil and shea butter. Transfer to a glass bowl. Add tea tree oil and whisk with an electric mixer for 1 minute, allow to cool for 20 minutes in refrigerator. Add your favorite essential oil. Whisk again until creamy and smooth. Store in an airtight container away from the sunlight or in the refrigerator.

Peppermint whipped body butter
Ingredients:
½ cup coconut oil
½ cup cocoa butter
½ cup shea butter
½ cut sweet almond oil
1 teaspoon vitamin E
2-4 drops peppermint essential oil
Method: In a double boiler, melt coconut oil, cocoa butter, and shea butter. Transfer to a glass bowl. Add sweet almond oil, vitamin E and peppermint oil. Mix together with electric blender for 5

minutes. Refrigerate for 20 minutes. Whisk again until creamy and soft. Store in an air tight container, away from the sunlight or in the refrigerator.

Lavender whipped body butter

Ingredients:

1-1/3 cups shea butter

½ cup extra virgin olive oil

1 teaspoon vitamin E

1 teaspoon rosemary oil extract

2 teaspoon lavender oil

Method: In a double boiler melt shea butter. Transfer to a glass bowl. Mix together shea butter, vitamin E, rosemary oil, and lavender oil. Mix well with a hand mixture until smooth and creamy.

Strawberry delight body butter

Ingredients:

2.5 tablespoons shea butter

1 teaspoon jojoba oil

1 teaspoon apricot oil

2 tablespoons coconut oil

¼ teaspoon strawberry food coloring

Few drops red food coloring

Method: In double boiler melt coconut and shea butters. Transfer to a glass bowl. Let cool for 30 minutes. Add jojoba and apricot oils. Whisk well. Add coloring and refrigerate for 20 minutes. After it is semi solid, blend with an electric mixer until smooth. Store in an airtight container away from the sunlight or in the refrigerator.

Ylang ylang sweet whipped body butter

Ingredients:

1 cup shea butter

½ cup coconut oil

½ cup sweet almond oil

10-30 drops ylang ylang

Method: In a double boiler melt shea butter, coconut oil and sweet almond oil. Once melted, remove from heat and cool slightly before adding essential oil. Place in refrigerator until mixture begins to harden. Mix with hand mixer until fluffy. Put into a clean container and return to refrigerator for about 10 minutes for mixture to set. Store in an air tight container, away from the sunlight or in the refrigerator.

Wild rose body butter
Rose absolute oil is calming and uplifting
Ingredients:
7 ounces shea butter
2 ounces sunflower oil
½ ounce Rosehip seed oil
8 drops rose absolute oil
10 drops geranium rose essential oil
½ teaspoon rose clay
2 teaspoons tapioca starch
Method: In double boiler melt shea butter and oils. Transfer to glass bowl. Add the rest of ingredients. Mix with a hand mixer until smooth and creamy. Store in an air tight container, away from the sunlight or in the refrigerator.

Frankincense whipped body butter
Ingredients:
½ cup extra virgin olive oil
½ cup shea butter
½ cup mango butter
1 ounce cocoa butter
1 teaspoon vitamin E
30 drops frankincense essential oil
Method: In a double boiler, melt shea butter mango butter and cocoa butter. Transfer to a glass bowl. Add olive oil. Let stand 15 minutes. Once cool, add vitamin E and frankincense essential oil. Cover bowl and refrigerate until semi-solid. Blend with an electric mixer until fluffy. Store in an air tight container, away from the sunlight or in the refrigerator.

Sugar Cookie Body Butter
Ingredients:
7 ounces liquid fractionated coconut oil
7 ounces cocoa butter

7 ounces shea butter
7 ounces sweet almond essential oil
4 drops tangerine essential oil
48 drops vanilla essential oil
4 drops cinnamon bark essential oil
2 drops ginger essential oil
Method: In a double boiler or microwave, melt together the cocoa butter, shea butter and sweet almond oil. Once completely melted, add in the liquid fractionated coconut oil. Allow the mixture to cool in the refrigerator for about 30 minutes or until it starts to harden. Using a mixer, whip the body butter for about 10 minutes to give it a nice fluffy texture. Add in the essential oils and continue to mix until the oils are fully incorporated into the body butter and the mixture has the consistency of cream. Put them into glass containers.

Moisturizing lemon eucalyptus body butter
Ingredients:
1 cup coconut oil
1 cup cocoa butter
10 drops lemon eucalyptus oil
1 cup almond oil
1 cup shea butter
Method: Melt all ingredients in a double boiler. Transfer to a glass bowl. Refrigerate until semi-hard. With electric mixer whisk until fluffy. Store in an air tight container, away from the sunlight or in the refrigerator.

Vanilla Cream Shea Butter
This shea butter vanilla cream is enriched with lavender essential oil and has an amazing natural scent. It is very quickly absorbed because there is no addition of other base oils. You can experiment with different quantities of vanilla and lavender to achieve a scent you prefer.

Ingredients:
2 ounces unrefined shea butter
5 drops lavender essential oil
5 drops vanilla essential oil
Method: Make sure unrefined shea butter is at room temperature

before you start. Mash it with a fork and add essential oils. Mash it again a little bit. Mix it with a hand mixer for a few minutes and you are done!

Rosemary mint shea body butter

Ingredients:

3 tablespoons cocoa butter

6 tablespoons shea butter

3 tablespoons extra virgin olive oil

20 drops spearmint essential oil

Method: Melt cocoa butter, shea butter, and extra virgin olive oil together in a double boiler. Transfer to a glass bowl. Let cool for 20 minutes in refrigerator. Whisk with electric mixer until it turns creamy white. Add spearmint essential oil and keep mixing until smooth and soft. Store in an air tight container, away from the sunlight or in the refrigerator.

Triple treat body butter

Ingredients:

1 cup coconut oil

½ cup shea butter

½ cup sweet almond oil

Method: In a double boiler, melt shea butter. Add coconut oil and stir. Add sweet almond oil. Place in the refrigerator to set 30 minutes until it is semi solid. Mix with a hand mixer until it forms a white peak. Refrigerate again for 20 minutes. Whip three more minutes. Refrigerate for another 10 minutes. Whip for 2 minutes more. Scoop into jars and allow to set at room temperature for 36 hours. Store in an air tight container, away from the sunlight or in the refrigerator.

Magnesium Body Butter

This magnesium body butter is wonderfully moisturizing and is great for helping your body relax.

Ingredients:

½ cup coconut oil

¼ cup shea butter

¼ cup cocoa butter

¼ cup magnesium topical spray (Nowfoods.com)

(optional) 10 to 20 drops lavender oil

Method: In a double boiler over low heat or in a microwave oven, melt the coconut oil with shea and cocoa butters. Pour into medium-sized bowl and let cool at room temperature for about 30 minutes, or until it begins to get cloudy. Using a mixer or blender, whip ingredients together, while slowly adding in the magnesium liquid. Place in the refrigerator for about 15-20 minutes or until oils are solid but still soft to the touch. Add in your desired drops of essential oil and re-blend to create a nice whip and fluffy texture. Place completed body butter into a glass jar or jars of your choosing with a tight seal. To Use: Spread onto skin to moisturize before bed. A little bit goes a long way. Relax and enjoy!

Raspberry vanilla body butter
Ingredients:
5-1/2 ounces cocoa butter
5-1/2 ounces shea butter
1.2 ounce grapeseed oil
2.5 ounces apricot kernel oil
2 drops vitamin E oil
.5 ounce black raspberry vanilla fragrance (Amazon)

Method: In double boiler melt oils and butters together. Transfer to a glass bowl. Add vitamin E and black raspberry vanilla fragrance. Mix well by hand. Refrigerate 20 minutes. Wisk thoroughly with an electric mixer until mixture is smooth creamy and soft. Store in an air tight container, away from the sunlight or in the refrigerator.

Shea Butter Cream for Extra Dry Skin
Ingredients:
1 and a half tablespoons of beeswax
1 tablespoon of kokum butter
2 tablespoons of coconut oil
1 tablespoon Shea butter
2 tablespoons of cocoa butter
8 drops sweet orange oil
1-½ tablespoons of rosehip oil

Method: In a double boiler, melt beeswax, kokum butter, coconut oil, shea butter and cocoa butter. Remove from heat and whip generously. Add sweet orange and rosehip oil and whip again.

Lavender Shea Butter Cream

Make this whipped body cream with beautiful texture in just a few minutes.

Ingredients:

4 ounces unrefined shea butter

2 tablespoons extra virgin olive oil

10-20 drops lavender essential oil

Method: Before you start, make sure your unrefined shea butter is room temperature. Do not melt or heat it! Put your shea butter in a mixing bowl and mash it with a fork. Add extra virgin olive oil and mash it a little bit more. Mix it on a high speed with electric mixer for approximately 5 minutes. Add lavender oil and mix it a few minutes to blend it into a whipped cream. Put whipped mixture in a clean jar(s) and close it. Keep it in a dry, and cool place. Room temperature is fine. There is no risk that your shea butter cream will become grainy, which sometimes happen in the case of melting. You can be sure all the temperature sensitive ingredients will be completely preserved.

Massage

Massage is good for the mind, body and soul.

Cooling and Soothing Neck and Body Massage

Massage this blend into your neck and shoulders, or overworked muscle groups in the legs or arms.

Ingredients:

1 cup shea butter

7 drops eucalyptus essential oil

4 drops peppermint essential oil

3 drops patchouli essential oil

Method: Melt shea butter in microwave. Add essential oils to melted shea butter. Mix well and apply as a massage to the back and sides of the neck and along the tops of your shoulders.

Sensuous Scented Butters

Creamy Sickle Scent for Kids

Ingredients:
2 tablespoons shea butter
4 drops vanilla essential oil
1 drop sweet orange essential oil
Method: Blend oils together in a small plastic container. Dab on the wrists, the neck, or behind the ears.

Patchouli Personal Essence

Patchouli oil helps create a peaceful and calming environment.

Ingredients:
½ cup shea butter
10 drops bergamot essential oil
4 drops rose essential oil
6 drops patchouli essential oil
Method: Melt shea butter in microwave. Combine all oils with shea butter and mix well.

Things are Just Rosey

Rose absolute oil is traditionally calming and uplifting also used for relieving stress.
Ingredients:
½ cup shea butter
1 drop of geranium oil
15 drops of rose absolute oil
Method: Make sure unrefined shea butter is at room temperature before you start. Mash it with a fork and add essential oils. Mash it again a little bit.

Blues Relief Cream

Ingredients:
2 drops clove oil
2 drops lemon essential oil
3 drops orange oil
2 ounces unrefined shea butter
Method: Make sure unrefined shea butter is at room temperature before you start. Mash it with a fork and add essential oils. Whip with hand mixer until creamy.

Hand Picked Passion

Jasmine essential oil has a rich, sultry aroma that makes this oil feel alluring and romantic.

Ingredients:

4 ounces unrefined shea butter

5 drops geranium oil

6 drops Jasmine absolute oil

Method: Make sure unrefined shea butter is at room temperature before you start. Mash it with a fork and add essential oils. Mash it again a little bit.

Goodnight Sleep

Ingredients:

2 drops of sage oil

1 drop of ylang ylang oil

20 drops of Neroli Blend Oil (nowfoods.com)

2 ounces unrefined shea butter

Method: Make sure unrefined shea butter is at room temperature before you start. Mash it with a fork and add essential oils. Whip with hand mixer until smooth and creamy.

Peace of Mind

Chamomile oil helps fight anxiety and depression and reduces symptoms of insomnia.

Ingredients:

10 drops of lavender oil

6 drops of chamomile oil

2 ounces unrefined shea butter

Method: Make sure unrefined shea butter is at room temperature before you start. Mash it with a fork and add essential oils. Whip with hand mixer until creamy.

Unwind Time

Sandalwood oil is a great stress reliever

Ingredients:

1 drop of chamomile oil

2 drops of lavender oil

2 drops of sandalwood oil

2 ounces unrefined shea butter

Method: Make sure unrefined shea butter is at room temperature before you start. Mash it with a fork and add essential oils. Whip with a hand mixer until the consistency is like butter.

Relaxing blend
Vanilla concentrate oil is sometimes used as an aphrodisiac.
Ingredients:
2 drops of Jasmine oil
2 drops of lavender oil
15 drops of vanilla concentrate oil
2 ounces unrefined shea butter
Method: Make sure unrefined shea butter is at room temperature before you start. Mash it with a fork and add essential oils. Whip with a hand mixer until the consistency is that of cream.

Daily Balance
Clary sage oil works as an effective natural remedy for depression.
Ingredients:
2 ounces unrefined shea butter
2 drops of geranium oil
2 drops of rose absolute oil
2 drops of clary sage oil
Method: Make sure unrefined shea butter is at room temperature before you start. Mash it with a fork and add essential oils. Whip with a hand mixer until the consistency is like butter.

Mental Focus body butter
Ingredients:
2 ounces unrefined shea butter
3 drops eucalyptus oil
2 drops peppermint oil
2 drops tangerine oil
Method: Make sure unrefined shea butter is at room temperature before you start. Mash it with a fork and add essential oils. Whip with a hand mixer until the consistency is like butter.

Cheer Up Buttercup Blend:
Ingredients:
1 drop of lime oil

1 drop grapefruit oil,
2 drops lemon oil
6 drops of tangerine oil
3 tablespoons shea butter
Method: Make sure unrefined shea butter is at room temperature before you start. Mash it with a fork and add essential oils. Whip with a hand mixer until the consistency is like butter.

Perfect Harmony body butter
Hyssop Essential Oil may be beneficial in the releasing and cleansing of negative emotions.
Ingredients:
3 ounces unrefined shea butter
2 drops of hyssop oil
2 drops of thyme oil
2 drops of bergamot oil
3 drops of chamomile oil
2 drops of neroli blend oil
Method: Make sure unrefined shea butter is at room temperature before you start. Mash it with a fork and add essential oils. Whip with a hand mixer until the consistency is like butter.

Botanical Bliss Body Butter
Ingredients:
3 ounces unrefined shea butter
5 drops rose absolute
2 drops ylang ylang oil
Method: Make sure unrefined shea butter is at room temperature before you start. Mash it with a fork and add essential oils. Whip with a hand mixer until the consistency is like butter.

Cloud 9 body butter
Ingredients:
2 ounces unrefined shea butter
1 drop of ylang ylang oil
1 drop of rose absolute oil
5 drops of patchouli oil
4 drops of sandalwood oil
Method: Make sure unrefined shea butter is at room temperature

before you start. Mash it with a fork and add essential oils. Whip with a hand mixer until the consistency is like butter.

Love is in the Air
Ingredients:
4 ounces unrefined shea butter
1 drop patchouli oil
3 drops jasmine oil
5 drops geranium oil
Method: Make sure unrefined shea butter is at room temperature before you start. Mash it with a fork and add essential oils. Whisk until creamy.

Tender Touch

Ingredients:

1 drop of ylang ylang oil

1 drop of bergamot oil

13 drops of Jasmine absolute oil

Method: Make sure unrefined shea butter is at room temperature before you start. Mash it with a fork and add essential oils. Whisk until creamy.

Calming Night

Ingredients:

4 drops of cypress oil

4 drops of lavender oil

4 drops of marjoram oil

2 ounces unrefined shea butter

Method: Make sure unrefined shea butter is at room temperature before you start. Mash it with a fork and add essential oils. Whip with hand blender until creamy.

Sweet peach body butter

Ingredients:

1 teaspoon honey

20 drops peach essential oil

½ cup shea butter

½ cup coconut oil

Method: In double boiler melt shea and coconut butters, Transfer to a glass bowl. Add peach essential oil and honey. Mix well until it is light and soft. Store in an air tight container, away from the sunlight or in the refrigerator.

Tropical mix body butter

Ingredients:

2-1/2 tablespoons cocoa butter

1 teaspoon vitamin E

1 teaspoon almond oil

20 drops citrus essential oil

3 tablespoons shea butter

1 tablespoon beeswax

Method: In a double boiler melt shea butter and beeswax.

Transfer into glass bowl. Let cool for 20 minutes. Add almond oil and vitamin E. Mix again. Add citrus essential oil. Mix until smooth. Store in an air tight container, away from the sunlight or in the refrigerator.

Raspberry vanilla body butter
Ingredients:
5-1/2 ounces cocoa butter
5-1/2 ounces shea butter
1.2 ounce grapeseed oil
2.5 ounces apricot kernel oil
2 drops vitamin E oil
.5 ounce black raspberry vanilla fragrance
Method: In double boiler melt oils and butters together. Transfer to a glass bowl. Add vitamin E and black raspberry vanilla fragrance. Mix well by hand. Refrigerate 20 minutes. Wisk thoroughly with an electric mixer until mixture is smooth creamy and soft. Store in an air tight container, away from the sunlight or in the refrigerator.

Peaceful Sleep Body Butter
Ingredients:
7 ounces coconut oil
7 ounces shea butter
7 ounces pure cocoa butter
7 ounces fractionated coconut oil
(optional) 10 to 20 drops Peaceful Sleep Oil Blend (Nowfoods.com)
Method: In a double boiler, combine cocoa butter, shea butter and coconut oil. Add in fractionated coconut oil. Allow the mixture to cool for about an hour or until it starts to harden (can be placed in fridge to speed up the process). Once the mixture is set, add in your desired drops of Peaceful Sleep Essential Oil Blend (start with fewer drops and add to your desired scent intensity). Use a hand mixer to whip the body butter for about 10 minutes to give it a nice, fluffy texture. Place completed body butter into a glass jar or jars of your choosing with a tight seal. Creates 32 total ounces (two 16 oz. containers). Spread onto skin to moisturize before bed. A little bit goes a long way. Relax and enjoy!

Silky gold body butter

Ingredients:

½ cup honey

2/3 cup shea butter

2 tablespoons wheat germ oil

2 teaspoons grapefruit seed extract

3 drops sandalwood essential oil

2 – 3 sheets 24 karat gold leaf (Amazon)

Method: In a double boiler melt wheat germ oil, honey, shea butter. Transfer the melted mixture into a glass bowl. Add the grapefruit seed extract and sandalwood. Blend thoroughly until fluffy. Crush the gold leaf and add to mixture. Mix again with a spatula. Store in an air tight container, away from the sunlight or in the refrigerator.

Exotic Nights Massage Butter

Ingredients:

2 ounces unrefined shea butter

3 drops orange oil

2 drops ylang ylang oil

Method: Make sure unrefined shea butter is at room temperature before you start. Mash it with a fork and add essential oils. Whip with a hand mixer until the consistency is like butter.

Muscle & Joint Soothing Massage Butter

Create this penetrating massage blend to soothe and restore sore, tired muscles after a long, hard day or vigorous workout.

Ingredients:

2 tablespoons sweet almond oil

2 tablespoons shea butter

3 drops lavender essential oil

3 drops peppermint essential oil

3 drops eucalyptus essential oil

Method: Combine all ingredients and mix well. Massage cream into muscles.

Mental Soothing body massage

Ingredients:

1 cup shea butter

5 drops rose otto essential oil
5 drops jasmine essential oil
2 drops lavender essential oil
1 drop sandalwood essential oil
1 drop vanilla essential oil
1 drop neroli essential oil
Method: Mix all ingredients together and use as a relaxing body massage.

Lovers Massage
Ingredients
1/2 cup shea butter
1 tablespoon grapeseed oil
1 tablespoon sweet almond or apricot kernel oil
10 drops rose absolute essential oil
7 drops sandalwood essential oil
Method: Melt shea butter at room temperature. Combine all ingredients and whip until creamy. Find a warm, cozy place free from interruptions and take turns massaging with your partner.

Mental Soothing body massage
Ingredients:
1 cup shea butter
5 drops rose otto essential oil
5 drops jasmine essential oil
2 drops lavender essential oil
1 drop sandalwood essential oil
1 drop vanilla essential oil
1 drop neroli essential oil
Method: Mix all ingredients together and use as a relaxing body massage.

Sweet Romance Massage butter
Ingredients:
4 ounces unrefined shea butter
2 drops cedarwood oil
2 drops clary sage oil
7 drops vanilla oil

1 drop orange oil

Method: Make sure unrefined shea butter is at room temperature before you start. Mash it with a fork and add essential oils. Whip with a hand mixer until the consistency is like butter.

Meditation Scents

Me time meditation butter

Ingredients:

2 ounces unrefined shea butter

1 drop sandalwood oil

2 drops clove oil

3 drops patchouli oil

Method: Make sure unrefined shea butter is at room temperature before you start. Mash it with a fork and add essential oils. Whip with a hand mixer until the consistency is like butter.

Floral Meditation

Ingredients:

2 ounces unrefined shea butter

5 drops rose absolute oil

1 drop geranium oil

Method: Make sure unrefined shea butter is at room temperature before you start. Mash it with a fork and add essential oils. Whip with a hand mixer until the consistency is like butter.

Body Scrubs

Blood Orange and Frankincense Whipped Shea Butter Oil Scrub

Ingredients:

3 tablespoons organic unrefined shea butter

24 drops blood orange essential oil

24 drops frankincense essential oil

5 tablespoons granulated sugar

Method: In a microwave, melt shea butter and remove. With a glass bowl let cool until just turning hazy. Add essential oils and sugar to shea butter. Set bowl in an ice bath and with a wire whisk, whip vigorously until creamy and firm, then transfer to wide-mouth jar. To use, apply to damp skin and scrub with gentle, circular motions. Rinse with warm water and pat dry.

Joint and Muscle Butters

Arthritis Rub
 Ingredients:
15 drops lavender oil
15 drops rosemary oil
Shea butter base
Contains just the right blend of three pain relieving oils (natural lavender, rosemary and shea butter) combined to relieve the pain of arthritis.

Known for its calming, relaxing and soothing effects, lavender is said to balance the central nervous system. Very valuable for all types of conditions involving spasms or pain such as rheumatism, arthritis, and muscular aches and pains.

Rosemary essential oil's anti-inflammatory qualities are known to relieve pain in headaches, muscle pain, rheumatism, and arthritis.

Natural Sunblock

Lavender Sunblock
Ingredients:
2 teaspoons virgin coconut oil
2 teaspoons organic shea butter
2 teaspoons vitamin E oil
1 teaspoon avocado oil
1 teaspoon sweet almond oil
6-8 drops lavender oil
Method: Melt the virgin coconut oil and organic shea butter in a double boiler. After melting, remove from heat and add vitamin E oil, avocado oil, sweet almond oil and mix together then add lavender essential oil. Allow to sit in fridge for about 35 minutes to partly

solidify. Mix well with hand mixer until creamy.

"Beauty is only skin deep."
Thomas Overbury

Cold and Flu Chest Rub

Basic Cold & Flu Chest Rub
Ingredients:
1 drop of lemon oil
2 drops of eucalyptus oil
1 drop of rosemary
1 tablespoon shea butter
Method: Mix ingredients together in a glass bowl and apply to chest and neck area. May also apply to forehead, cheekbone and nose areas, discontinue use if irritation occurs.

Stretch Marks

How beautiful do you feel when you're pregnant? All that stuff about how beautiful a pregnant woman is was obviously written by men! Take all the beauty treatments and tips in this guide, multiply them by three and maybe, just maybe we might feel a little bit better about how we look and feel. Massage shea butter cream on stretch marks to help fade them away.

Smoothing Butter
Ingredients:
4 ounces natural shea butter
1 capsule vitamin E
Add your favorite essential oil scents
Method: Using shea butter as a carrier, mix a few drops of your favorite essential oils. Always use shea butter for the ultimate softening of the skin.

Cocoa and Shea Butter Stretch Marks Remover
Ingredients:
2 tablespoons coconut oil

2 tablespoons cocoa butter
2 tablespoons shea butter
1 tablespoon avocado oil
Few drops of vitamin E
Add any aromatic essential oil for fragrance
Method: Place the ingredients in the top of a double boiler and melt on low heat. Use a hand mixer to whip the body butter for about 10 minutes to give it a nice fluffy texture. Place completed body butter into a glass jar or jars of your choosing with a tight seal.

Body Lotion for Stretch Marks
Ingredients:
½ cup almond or olive oil
¼ cup fractionated coconut oil
¼ cup beeswax
2 tablespoons shea or cocoa butter
Essential oil, (vanilla or other)
Method: Combine ingredients in a pint jar. Fill medium saucepan with a couple inches of water and place over medium heat. Put a lid on the jar loosely and place in the pan with the water. As the water heats, the ingredients in the jar will start to melt. Shake or stir occasionally to incorporate. When all ingredients are completely melted, pour into tin or jar. Let cool completely and massage over stretch marks.

Cellulite attack cinnamon body butter
Ingredients:
3.5 ounces coconut oil
1.5 ounces cocoa butter
1.5 ounces shea butter
30 drops cinnamon oil
1 cinnamon stick
Method: In double boiler, melt cocoa butter, coconut oil and shea butter together. Transfer to a glass bowl. Let cool for 20 minutes. Add cinnamon oil. Mix with a hand mixer until creamy and smooth. Break the cinnamon stick into small pieces and add to the soft mixture. Store in an airtight container, away from the sunlight or in the refrigerator.

Body Shaving Cream

Ingredients:

¼ cup coconut oil

2-3 tablespoons shea butter

¼ cup aloe vera gel

2 tablespoons baking soda

¼ cup liquid castile soap

a few drops of vitamin E

5-10 drops essential oil

Method: Combine coconut oil and shea butter in a double boiler until just melted. Remove from heat and mix in other ingredients. Place in fridge for 30 minutes until top and sides start to solidify. Using an electric mixer, blend well for 5-8 minutes. Mixture should be fluffy like whipped cream, but denser. Transfer to air tight jar.

BATHING BEAUTY

Happiness is a hot bubble bath

Whether or not a bath should be taken at night or in the morning is a question which each person must decide for him or herself. While it has often been said that a bath at night will quiet the nerves and make you sleep soundly, there have been persons who found that a bath at night caused them to be restless and wide awake.

One reason why a bath before going to bed is desirable, is that a soothing body butter can be applied to the face, neck and hands leaving the skin soft and beautiful. After a warm bath, the pores of the skin are opened and in excellent condition to absorb a good natural skin cream.

A course complexion with black disfiguring open pores can be almost entirely cured by keeping the pores of the body free from dirt. To be extra clean, each day, have the bathtub carefully scoured as the oils and dirt washed from the body invariably collect on the sides of the tub where the water has reached.

Dry yourself quickly then put on a warm robe while the hair is being combed for the night, the teeth brushed, and the face massaged with a pure home-made face cream. Then go to bed and you will find a prettier, fresher complexion when you awaken the next morning.

Well this is the time to use your delicious shea butter recipe for smoothing and softening the body. It's nice to go to bed with a body softened by shea butter, but it's even nicer to go to bed with a body softened by sensuous shea butter. It not only softens your skin but soothes your mind with a calming aroma.

Coconut Cocoa Shea Balm

Ingredients:

3 tablespoons coconut oil

1 tablespoon cocoa butter

4 tablespoons shea butter

20 drops sweet orange oil

Method: In a double boiler or microwave, warm coconut oil, shea butter and cocoa butter. Remove from heat and let cool. Add sweet orange oil and whip with a hand mixer until creamy.

Hefty muscle balm

Ingredients:

½ cup coconut oil

3 tablespoons beeswax pastilles

2 tablespoons shea butter

½ teaspoon vitamin E

20 drops lavender essential oil

Method: In a double boiler, melt coconut oil, beeswax, shea butter, vitamin E. Stir. Remove from heat. Add lavender oil. Pour into a container.

Moisturizing Bath Salt

Ingredients:

¼ cup sea salt

¼ cup Epsom salt

3-6 drops essential oil (your choice of fragrance)

1 tablespoon sweet almond oil

2 tablespoons shea butter

Method: Mix all ingredients together. Stir until well mixed. Add 2 tablespoons Moisturizing bath salts to your bath while water is running. Sit back and enjoy.

NATURAL DEODORANTS

Nature's New Magic

Deodorants are a hot topic these days. There are major concerns of the link between aluminum in deodorants and Alzheimer's, as well as the threat of Parabens causing cancer. The research has shown conflicting results, but just the idea of such risks is frightening.

It's been told that there is aluminum in your deodorant and it's been linked to breast cancer and Alzheimer's disease. Who wants that? But if you want deodorant that does not include aluminum, here are a few recipes to help you make your own. It turns out awesome and it is so easy. You probably have all the ingredients at home anyway and won't have to spend any extra money at the store. Bonus! Your pits have never smelled better!

We all know that shea butter has the power of rejuvenating the skin and lemon juice can be used for weight loss, but did you know that these two natural ingredients can be used together to produce a great natural deodorant?

The recipe is simple. All you need is one teaspoon of shea butter and a squirt of fresh lemon or lime juice mixed in a small cup.

Because lemon juice is very acidic and may burn your skin and often drying it out, shea butter combines beautifully with it for a gentler interaction with your skin. The citrus smell of lemon combined with the natural musk of shea butter leaves you feeling confident and makes others happy to be around you as well. The lightening effect of lemon juice is great in toning dark or discolored armpits leaving you ready to sport your lovely sleeveless outfits.

With these recipes you not only smell good, but your skin stays pampered and naturally cared for giving you an extra confidence boost and saving you quite a bit of money. It's also a healthier alternative in the long run to other products full of laboratory chemicals that can't be fully accounted for and which have been blamed for skin ailments and inconsistencies.

Lemony Shea Deodorant
Ingredients:
1 teaspoon natural shea butter
1 squirt of fresh lemon juice
(Leftovers can be kept refrigerated for 3 days)

Deodorant for Sensitive Skin
Ingredients:
1 tablespoon coconut oil
1-1/2 tablespoons beeswax (grated)
1 tablespoon shea butter
4 teaspoons bentonite clay
20 drops essential oil (lavender and rosemary)
Method: Melt coconut oil and beeswax in a double boiler. Add shea butter and whisk for 2 minutes. Remove from heat and add clay – whisk again. Finally add essential oil and stir. Let cool. Spoon into deodorant container

Tea Tree Deodorant
Ingredients:
1/4 cup organic coconut oil
1/4 cup aluminum-free baking soda
1/4 cup arrowroot powder
16 drops of tea tree or lavender essential oil
Method: Slightly melt coconut oil just until soft and not clumpy. Then mix everything else in a bowl and combine. Store in a 4 oz Jar. Apply with your fingers and that's it. Also, if you have sensitive skin, use less baking soda.

Cocoa butter Deodorant
Ingredients:
3 tablespoons shea butter
3 tablespoons aluminum free baking soda
2 tablespoons corn starch
2 tablespoons cocoa butter

2 vitamin E oil gel caps (puncture and squeeze out the oil)
ylang ylang and orange essential oil

Melt all the ingredients (except the Vitamin E and essential oils) and stir well. Then add the oils and stir again. Pour the mixture into a ¼ pint jar and place in the refrigerator until it hardens. The deodorant goes on white-ish and gets clear-ish later. It does not prevent sweating but does a great job of eliminating any bad odor, and adds a nice, fresh smell.

Beeswax and Clay deodorant

Ingredients:
1.5 tablespoons beeswax
4 tablespoons shea butter
1 tablespoon cocoa butter
4 teaspoons bentonite or kaolin clay
20-25 drops tea tree essential oil

Method: Measure the beeswax, cocoa butter and shea butter into a microwavable container. Pop it into the microwave and microwave on high for 1-3 minutes, or until the mixture is mostly melted. Stir to finish melting everything down into a clear liquid. You can let it cool over night at room temperature or after 15 minutes, pop into the freezer for about 30 minutes. Either way, when it's all cooled off and room temp, cap it up and use lightly as needed.

NOTES: Keep away from heat and warm light (sunlight). Leave it on a dresser top that's always in the shade and not in your hot bathroom. You don't want to have your deodorant melt away.

You know exactly what's in your homemade deodorant. It's not a secret.

Coconut Oil: Softens, but especially adds extra antibacterial protection. Bacteria is what leads to stinkiness. Coconut oil is your best weapon.

Shea Butter: Softens (a lot). It will also most likely help with the little bumps you get from shaving.

Clay: Adds extra dryness protection. It will help at whisking away sweat and drying it up before it reaches your clothes. However, don't expect it to work quite as well as antiperspirant (which contains the aluminum you REALLY want to avoid). They work in two very different ways.

Beeswax: This may help, a little, with the perspiration problem, but the main point of this ingredient is to give the deodorant a more solid feel, so it'll stay in your container the way you want it to.

Tea Tree and/or Rosemary Essential Oil: These two oils are exceptionally antibacterial and antifungal, so they'll work hard at keeping any stinkiness from happening. Again, you can use any essential oil you'd like for scent (lavender, bergamot and lemon essential oils would be great as a substitution for tea tree and rosemary in terms of odor-stopping).

Sweet Orange & Frankincense Deodorant

This recipe makes a cream style natural deodorant that you store in a jar and spread on with your fingers. You only need a small amount to be effective!

Herbal Infused Coconut Oil for Skin Soothing Benefits

To add an extra boost of goodness to your homemade deodorant, try infusing the coconut oil with herbs before making this deodorant.

Ingredients:
1 ounce (28 g) shea butter
1 ounce (28 g) beeswax
2 ounces (57 g) coconut oil
1 tablespoon baking soda (or bentonite clay)
1 tablespoon arrowroot powder
1/4 teaspoon (about 24 drops) sweet orange essential oil
4 to 6 drops frankincense essential oil
Method: In a double boiler, melt the shea butter, beeswax and coconut oil. Remove from heat. Stir in the baking soda or clay, arrowroot powder and essential oils. Stir frequently while cooling to ensure a creamy texture. Spoon the finished deodorant in a jar. This recipe almost fills a 4 ounce jar. Shelf life is around 9 months to 1 year. Keep out of direct sunlight and store in a cool dry area.

Troubleshooting

If your deodorant turns out too hard for your preference, melt it again and add a teaspoon or two of a liquid oil such as jojoba, sunflower, sweet almond, etc.

If the deodorant is too soft, try melting it and adding a pinch more beeswax.

Make sure to stir, stir, stir, especially in the first 5 to 10 minutes that the deodorant is cooling. This is what gives it a creamier texture.

If your deodorant develops graininess over time, that's likely from the shea butter. To fix, melt the batch of deodorant until entirely melted and no lumps remain. Stir well as it cools. You may need to add a few more drops of essential oil in case some of the scent evaporates during reheating.

Remember that homemade deodorants help with odor protection, but they don't act as antiperspirants. You will still sweat when using homemade deodorant.

Coconut Shea Deodorant
1-1/2 tablespoons grated beeswax or beeswax beads
4 tablespoons coconut oil
1 tablespoon shea butter
4 teaspoons clay (bentonite or other)
20-25 drops essential oil (tea tree, rosemary, lavender, lemon, bergamot, or a mixture of any listed)
Empty, clean, sterilized deodorant container
Method: Melt the beeswax and coconut oil on very low heat, whisking often. Once melted, add in the shea butter and whisk a few times, then remove from the heat and continue melting. After that's melted and you have a liquid, sprinkle in the clay and continue to whisk well until everything is combined. Drop in the essential oil, whisking still. Place the pan into a cool water bath and leave for 5 minutes or until it just begins to set up. Spoon the mixture into your deodorant container and place it in the freezer for 20-30 minutes (or until completely hard. If, for some reason, it starts to get too soft on a hot day, just put it back in the freezer for a while.

FANCY FEET

Beauty Tips for Flattering Feet

You jam your feet into fashionable shoes, kick them around, stub their toes, ignore their nails and demand that they carry you around all day. No wonder they look a little worse for the wear. Luckily, there are plenty of simple, inexpensive tricks you can use to have your feet looking and feeling their best in no time at all.

There are so many features of everyday living that are absolutely torturous for your feet. Standing all day, too-small shoes, stuffy boots, and exposing them to the locker room floor at your local gym are examples of scenarios to which most women can relate. Feet are often taken for granted until they start to hurt and reject the burdens you place on them, so think of taking care of your feet now as an investment against problems in the future.

Use a dollop of your own home-made shea butter foot cream to soften any rough spots like your heels or the sides of your toes. Once you've massaged your hand made cream into your feet, put on a pair of socks (preferably silk socks from Amazon) and relax for the night.

That's it! You're ready to strap on a pair of open-toe sandals or pad around the house in your bare, and very fashionable, flattering feet.

Looking pretty is one element of great feet. The other part is keeping your feet healthy. Wear supportive, well-fitted shoes, and wash and dry your feet carefully to avoid fungal and bacterial problems.

When it comes to skin care, the feet are often neglected. So, at bedtime, soak your feet for about fifteen minutes. Then, rinse them off and dry your feet well. And, add some homemade shea butter cream to your feet for an easy and quick fix pedicure.

Now here is another easy way to achieve soft and smooth feet at home without visiting a salon for an expensive and sometimes risky pedicure. Shea butter plus clean socks bring relief to dry, rough, callused feet. Use, your own homemade shea butter cream, and then slip on a pair of clean silk socks. Wearing socks work with the skin to help absorb and retain the valuable active oils that keep feet looking and feeling soft and smooth. Keep the socks on at least one hour or preferably overnight after applying your homemade shea butter foot cream.

Self-Treatment Foot Massage

Try a foot massage. It's relaxing and rejuvenating. Massage your feet yourself or ask your partner and trade off. Everyone wins! Here is how you can give an awesome foot massage to your special someone!

Sit down and begin to apply foot cream. Use a quarter size dollop of the foot cream on each foot. Keep most of the cream on the bottom of the feet and massage well into the heel or more calloused area of the foot. Massage into each foot a minute or two and then put a sock on. The sock should be worn about 1 hour but leaving it on overnight works best.

1. Prepare your surroundings. Get a folded towel to keep the foot cream from getting on your sheets or furniture while you work. Do what you wish to make the room relaxing: Light a candle, play some soft music, and have your shea butter foot cream at hand.

2. Use gliding strokes, and then kneading strokes: Place your thumbs in the bottom of your foot and apply slight pressure. Your other fingers should be on the top of the foot. See that group of mounds right before the front of the foot? Glide your thumbs right under them towards the toes. Once the foot is more relaxed, go on and knead. You want to see the foot move around a little.

3. Small Circles: Using small, slow circles, work your way around the heel. Heels take a lot of our pressure, so don't leave them out!

4. Use Squeezing and Wringing Strokes: Place both of your hands next to each other, gently squeezing the instep of the foot. Then slowly begin to move each hand in the opposite direction, like you're wringing out a wet wash cloth. Work using this wringing stroke from the heel up to the toes.

5. Use Gentle Stretches: Hold the heel with your left hand and cross your right hand to grab the instep. Give the foot a gentle stretch. Switch hands—right hand on heel and left hand on the outside of the foot—and repeat. Deep pressure isn't needed, and instead of tiring out your hands try to get most of your strength from rocking back and forth. You're on your way to giving a great massage!

6. Watch your speed and pressure. Remember: Slow and steady wins the race. A massage that's too vigorous is oftentimes the least relaxing.

If your ankles and feet are swelling, it's a sure sign you are holding fluids. Try to avoid sitting for long periods at a time and cut down on your salt intake.

Stilettos are beautiful and yes, they do make you look sexy, HOWEVER, you should avoid long walks while wearing them.

In fact, you should always wear sensible shoes. Ha! Fat chance, right? Seriously, what about a compromise? Wear sensible shoes when you are coming and/or going from work and keep the heels in a tote bag.

For extremely dry feet,

Lather on a layer of your shea butter foot cream to each foot; slip your feet into a pair of socks. Leave on overnight while sleeping and when you awaken the next morning your feet will feel smooth, silky and soft.

Rejuvenating Foot Cream

Ingredients:

4 ounces shea butter (room temperature)

2 tablespoons extra virgin olive oil

10 – 20 drops of lavender, sweet orange or peppermint essential oil

Method: Mash shea butter with a fork. Add extra virgin olive oil and mash some more. Put into a mixing bowl and mix on high speed for approximately 5 minutes. Add essential oils and mix for 5 minutes more.

Healing Foot Butter

Ingredients:

2 tablespoons Shea butter

2 tablespoons coconut oil

1 tablespoon grated cocoa butter

1 tablespoon plus 1 teaspoon grated beeswax

4 tablespoons jojoba oil

30 drops lavender essential oil (optional)

Makes approximately 4 ounces

Super for dry, cracked and damaged skin.

Method: Mash shea butter with a fork. Add oils and mash some more. Put in mixing bowl and mix on high speed for approximately 5 minutes. Add essential oils and mix for 5 minutes more.

Nature's Soothing Foot Scrub

Ingredients:

3 tablespoons of shea butter

1/4 teaspoon extra virgin olive oil

½ teaspoon castile soap

1 teaspoon dried lemon peel

Method: Mix together and use as a natural foot scrub.

Menthol Foot Butter

Ingredients:

1.5 ounces shea Butter

0.5 ounce cocoa butter

0.5 ounce menthol crystals

20 drops rosemary essential oil
20 drops fir essential oil
10 drops lavender essential oil
10 drops tea tree essential oil

Method: Melt shea Butter in the top of a double boiler. Put the melted butter into a mixing bowl and grab your electric beaters. Blend it up a bit, until it's whippy and creamy. Weigh the cocoa butter and menthol crystals into a small heat resistant glass measuring cup and melt them together over a double boiler (menthol crystals are oil soluble). Pour the melted cocoa/menthol mixture over the shea Butter and whip the mixture together. Blend in the essential oils. Keep coming back to the mixture and whip it for a minute or so until it's set up nicely. Scoop your lovely foot butter into a 4 ounces wide-mouthed jar and enjoy!

Cooling foot cream

After a therapeutic soak and scrub, rinse feet well and follow up with a delightful foot massage using this cooling cream.

Ingredients:
1/2 ounce melted shea butter
4 ounces sweet almond oil or 3 ounces chamomile tea
3 ounces warm mint tea or 3 ounces warm chamomile tea
21 drops lavender essential oil
9 drops peppermint essential oil
6 drops spearmint essential oil

Method: Melt the shea butter and almond oil together in a microwave. Add the warm tea to the butter and oil mixture in a thin stream, whisking vigorously. Immerse the bowl in a cool water bath to make the cream congeal, again whisking vigorously. As the cream begins to form, add the essential oils, drop by drop, and whisk them into the mixture.

Make your feet take your where your

heart wants to go.

LOVE YOURSELF ALWAYS

Last but not least, learn to love yourself.

- Take a walk on the beach, in a forest or around the block.
- Get a collagen boost. Eat more fruit!
- Get enough exercise.
- Take time for hobbies or other activities. All work and no play will make Jane a dull girl or John very boring!
- Limit your red meat intake and eat more fish and fowl.
- Focus on the positive and if you falter, think about all the good things you've done.
- Laugh a lot. Remember what they say . . . it takes more muscles to frown than to laugh.
- Surround yourself with scents. Put an aromatherapy candle in the kitchen and another in the living room.
- Use a few drops of your favorite essential oil in your next bath.
- Be kind.
- Learn something new.

You're always one decision away from a totally different life.

CONCLUSION

If you want to start feeling and looking young, you have to make that step today. Each day that you wait to make a move is a day less to your goal of getting that wholesome beauty in your life.

Start now to incorporate positive and natural things into your life. You really have to work on looking young and beautiful.

The old lifestyle that you have dealt with in the past have to disappear. The new you will become more youthful and healthier. There are too many things out there that can destroy your youthfulness if you allow them. Take charge of your life and seek the new younger you today

.

ABOUT THE AUTHOR

I want to say "thank you" from the bottom of my heart for purchasing this book. I wrote this book for the beautiful people who wish to maintain their beauty without the use of harmful chemicals. Not only are you saving the environment, but you are also saving your body.

For many years I have been a naturalist. I believe that beauty can be achieved from the inside as well as from the outside and can be done chemical free. Therefore, for this reason I have researched recipes that will help you achieve a more beautiful and healthy life.

If you enjoyed this book, then please take a moment to leave a review. This valuable feedback will allow me to write e-books that help you in your journey through life. And if you love it, please let me know.